Lumen-Apposing Stents

Editor

JACQUES VAN DAM

GASTROINTESTINAL ENDOSCOPY CLINICS OF NORTH AMERICA

www.giendo.theclinics.com

Consulting Editor
CHARLES J. LIGHTDALE

April 2018 • Volume 28 • Number 2

ELSEVIER

1600 John F. Kennedy Boulevard • Suite 1800 • Philadelphia, Pennsylvania, 19103-2899

http://www.theclinics.com

GASTROINTESTINAL ENDOSCOPY CLINICS OF NORTH AMERICA Volume 28, Number 2
April 2018 ISSN 1052-5157, ISBN-13: 978-0-323-58306-0

Editor: Kerry Holland
Developmental Editor: Donald Mumford

Gastrointestinal Endoscopy Clinics of North America (ISSN 1052-5157) is published quarterly by Elsevier Inc., 360 Park Avenue South, New York, NY 10010-1710. Months of issue are January, April, July, and October. Business and Editorial Offices: 1600 John F. Kennedy Blvd., Suite 1800, Philadelphia, PA, 19103-2899. Periodicals postage paid at New York, NY and additional mailing offices. Subscription prices are $349.00 per year for US individuals, $593.00 per year for US institutions, $100.00 per year for US students and residents, $385.00 per year for Canadian individuals, $702.00 per year for Canadian institutions, $474.00 per year for international individuals, $702.00 per year for international institutions, and $245.00 per year for Canadian and foreign students/residents. To receive student/resident rate, orders must be accompanied by name of affiliated institution, date of term, and the *signature* of program/residency coordinator on institution letterhead. Orders will be billed at individual rate until proof of status is received. Foreign air speed delivery is included in all *Clinics* subscription prices. All prices are subject to change without notice. **POSTMASTER:** Send address change to *Gastrointestinal Endoscopy Clinics of North America*, Elsevier Health Sciences Division, Subscription Customer Service, 3251 Riverport Lane, Maryland Heights, MO 63043. **Customer Service: 1-800-654-2452 (US). From outside the United States, call 1-314-447-8871. Fax: 1-314-447-8029. E-mail: JournalsCustomerService-usa@elsevier.com (for print support) or JournalsOnlineSupport-usa@elsevier.com (for online support).**

Reprints. For copies of 100 or more, of articles in this publication, please contact the Commercial Reprints Department, Elsevier Inc., 360 Park Avenue South, New York, NY 10010-1710. Tel. 212-633-3874; Fax: 212-633-3820; E-mail: reprints@elsevier.com.

Gastrointestinal Endoscopy Clinics of North America is covered in *Excerpta Medica, MEDLINE/PubMed (Index Medicus), and MEDLINE/MEDLARS.*

Contributors

CONSULTING EDITOR

CHARLES J. LIGHTDALE, MD
Professor of Medicine, Division of Digestive and Liver Diseases, Columbia University
Medical Center, New York, New York, USA

EDITOR

JACQUES VAN DAM, MD, PhD
Professor of Medicine, Keck School of Medicine of USC, Los Angeles, California, USA

AUTHORS

SOPHOCLIS P. ALEXOPOULOS, MD, FACS
Associate Professor, Department of Surgery, Vanderbilt University, Nashville, Tennessee,
USA

STUART K. AMATEAU, MD, PhD
Director of Endoscopy, Assistant Professor, Department of Medicine, Division of
Gastroenterology, Hepatology and Nutrition, University of Minnesota, Minneapolis,
Minnesota, USA

JI YOUNG BANG, MD, MPH
Center for Interventional Endoscopy, Florida Hospital Orlando, Orlando, Florida, USA

TODD H. BARON, MD
Professor of Medicine, Division of Gastroenterology and Hepatology, The University of
North Carolina at Chapel Hill, Chapel Hill, North Carolina, USA

KENNETH F. BINMOELLER, MD
Director, Interventional Endoscopy Services, California Pacific Medical Center, California,
San Francisco, USA

BRIAN R. BOULAY, MD, MPH
Associate Professor of Clinical Medicine, Division of Gastroenterology and Hepatology,
University of Illinois Hospital & Health Sciences System, Chicago, Illinois, USA

JACK BRAHA, MD
Chief, Division of Gastroenterology, Mount Sinai Brooklyn, Greater New York Endoscopy
Surgical Center, Brooklyn, New York, USA

JAEHOON CHO, MD
Internal Medicine Resident, Department of Internal Medicine, LAC + USC Medical Center,
Los Angeles, California, USA

MARTIN L. FREEMAN, MD
Professor and Chief, Department of Medicine, Division of Gastroenterology, Hepatology and Nutrition, University of Minnesota, Minneapolis, Minnesota, USA

MARC GIOVANNINI, MD
Chief of Endoscopic Unit, Institute Paoli-Calmettes, Marseilles, France

MICHEL KAHALEH, MD, AGAF, FACG, FASGE
Division of Gastroenterology and Hepatology, NewYork-Presbyterian/Weill Cornell Medical Center, New York, New York, USA

RYAN LAW, DO
Assistant Professor of Medicine, Division of Gastroenterology, University of Michigan, Ann Arbor, Michigan, USA

SIMON K. LO, MD, FACP
Director, Pancreatic and Biliary Disease Program, F Widjaja Family Chair, Digestive Diseases, Cedars-Sinai Medical Center, Los Angeles, California, USA

LEA MATSUOKA, MD, FACS
Associate Professor, Department of Surgery, Vanderbilt University, Nashville, Tennessee, USA

ANDREW NETT, MD
Interventional Endoscopy Services, California Pacific Medical Center, California, San Francisco, USA

ARA B. SAHAKIAN, MD
Assistant Professor of Medicine, Division of Gastrointestinal and Liver Diseases, Keck School of Medicine of USC, Los Angeles, California, USA

MONICA SAUMOY, MD, MS
Division of Gastroenterology and Hepatology, NewYork-Presbyterian/Weill Cornell Medical Center, New York, New York, USA

MATTHEW W. STIER, MD
Gastroenterology Fellow, Center for Endoscopic Research and Therapeutics (CERT), The University of Chicago Medicine, Chicago, Illinois, USA

SCOTT TENNER, MD, MPH, FACG, FASGE, AGAF
Professor of Medicine, State University of New York, Director, Greater New York Endoscopy Surgical Center, Brooklyn, New York, USA

SHYAM VARADARAJULU, MD
Medical Director, Center for Interventional Endoscopy, Florida Hospital Orlando, Orlando, Florida, USA

IRVING WAXMAN, MD
Sara and Harold Lincoln Thompson Professor of Medicine and Surgery, Center for Endoscopic Research and Therapeutics (CERT), The University of Chicago Medicine, Chicago, Illinois, USA

CLARK YARBER
Central Michigan University, College of Medicine, Mount Pleasant, Michigan, USA

Contents

> Pseudocysts evolve from fluid collections and/or disruptions of the pancreatic duct. They may occur secondary to acute pancreatitis, pancreatic trauma, or chronic pancreatitis. Without the clinical information, radiologists may inappropriately call a fluid collection or any cystic lesion a pseudocyst. With no clear history of acute pancreatitis or chronic pancreatitis, this is rare. Complications include infection, intracystic hemorrhage, or rupture. Pseudocysts can become painful, especially with chronic pancreatitis, and can cause early satiety and weight loss when their size affects the stomach and bowel. Symptomatic pseudocysts can successfully be drained via surgical, radiologic, or endoscopic drainage.

> Open surgical intervention for the treatment of simple pancreatic pseudocyst (PP) has a high success rate and has been the historical gold standard. Open surgical intervention, however, confers significant morbidity and mortality, which has spurred the development of less invasive techniques. Laparoscopic approaches are feasible, with the potential for lower complication rates and length of stay. The endoscopic approach has the appeal of potentially shorter hospitalization length of stays and does not require general anesthesia. Complicated PPs or those that arise in the setting of chronic pancreatitis warrant additional workup and special consideration.

> Necessity is the mother of invention. The development of the lumen-apposing metal stent (LAMS) and "hot" electrocautery-enhanced delivery system marks the most recent evolutionary stage of endoscopic therapy of pancreatic fluid collections. It was conceived by the inventor to address limitations of the existing off-the-shelf tools available to endoscopists. The LAMS is the first stent specifically designed for endoscopic ultrasound-guided transluminal drainage of extraintestinal fluid collections. The impetus behind the LAMS and its delivery platform was to make

Future applications of the LAMS are continuously being developed as clinicians provide minimally invasive approaches for the management of these disease processes.

Matthew W. Stier and Irving Waxman

Numerous lumen-apposing metal stents (LAMSs) have been designed for transluminal applications, including complex pancreatic fluid collections (PFCs) and difficult biliary access. Limited high-quality data exist directly comparing the various LAMS models, and their use remains largely dependent on availability and operator expertise. LAMS placement has been streamlined by the addition of electrocautery, allowing for a single-step or modified "hot" approach, if desired. Therapeutic endoscopists continue to explore the application of this technology in a variety of clinical scenarios, and future innovations will be needed to meet these evolving clinical demands.

Stuart K. Amateau and Martin L. Freeman

The lumen-apposing metal stent has evolved endoscopic transluminal therapies, although it has potential complications, including maldeployment, bleeding, perforation, migration, and several risks specific to necrotizing pancreatitis. Careful planning and technique mitigate these inherent risks of lumen-apposing metal sent deployment; however, setbacks occur even in the most experienced of hands. Therefore, early recognition and management of these complications are critical to alleviating morbidity and avoiding mortality. Management frequently requires multidisciplinary effort, including advanced endoscopic technique and consultation of interventional radiologic and surgical colleagues.

Jaehoon Cho and Ara B. Sahakian

The development of new endoscopic techniques, such as gastrointestinal (GI) stenting, full-thickness suturing, clip application, and use of tissue adhesives, has had a significant impact on the management of GI fistulae. These techniques have shown promising results, but further study is needed to optimize the efficacy of long-term closure. The advancement of endoscopic techniques, including the use of the lumen-apposing metal stent (LAMS), has allowed for the deliberate creation of fistula tracts to apply endoscopic therapy that previously could not be achieved. This article examines the rapidly evolving area of endoscopic fistula closure and its relationship to LAMS.

Ji Young Bang and Shyam Varadarajulu

Lumen-apposing metal stents are integrated in a single-step delivery system for draining intraabdominal fluid collections. The theoretic advantage of lumen-apposing stents is the ability to approximate the wall of the drained cavity or organ to the gastrointestinal tract lumen. The use of lumen-apposing stents now includes drainage of organs adjacent to the stomach/duodenum and creation of anastomosis between the stomach and jejunum. The lumen-apposing stents may also serve as a conduit for accessing the remnant stomach for performing biliary tract interventions. This article outlines the approach to placement of lumen-apposing metal stents, technical challenges, and measures to counter adverse events.

GASTROINTESTINAL ENDOSCOPY CLINICS OF NORTH AMERICA

THE CLINICS ARE AVAILABLE ONLINE!
Access your subscription at:
www.theclinics.com

Foreword

Lumen-Apposing Metal Stents: An Important New Tool for Interventional Endoscopy Comes of Age

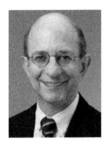

Charles J. Lightdale, MD
Consulting Editor

Brilliant is the word that comes to mind. Lumen-apposing metal stents (LAMS) that are placed through an endoscope can connect separate gastrointestinal (GI) structures. LAMS can safely accomplish in a minimally invasive manner what could only be done previously through surgical incisions. The accumulating results show tremendous benefits for patients. The key to this success was the revolutionary invention of linear array endoscopic ultrasound (EUS). These instruments allowed real-time visualization through the lumen of the GI tract organ containing the endoscope and further out to image an adjacent lumen. The EUS technology then allowed a needle to be placed accurately under ultrasound guidance through the endoscopic lumen into the adjacent lumen, and through the needle a guide wire, and over the wire a stent. All pretty neat and classical interventional radiology stuff, but with minimal fluoroscopy. The genius part was the LAMS, an amazing combination of metallurgy and engineering that brings the two lumens together leaving an opening between them through the stent, but preventing GI contents from leaking into the peritoneal cavity.

The Editor for this issue of *Gastrointestinal Endoscopy Clinics of North America* is Dr Jacques Van Dam, an inventive leader in interventional endoscopy. He has assembled a remarkable group of endoscopic pioneer authors, producing a state-of-the-art review of LAMS. The first four articles focus on pancreatic pseudocysts and fluid collections, where LAMS have had the greatest use to date, followed by articles on biliary and gallbladder drainage, a growing area for LAMS, followed by an article on other novel and promising uses. Importantly, there are articles on complications: how to avoid them and how to manage them. Finally, there are practical topics on selection

Gastrointest Endoscopy Clin N Am 28 (2018) xi–xii
https://doi.org/10.1016/j.giec.2018.01.002
1052-5157/18/© 2018 Published by Elsevier Inc.

of which LAMS to utilize in different clinical situations and a step-by-step description of how to perform a LAMS procedure. This is altogether a terrific issue of *Gastrointestinal Endoscopy Clinics of North America* that should be widely appreciated.

Charles J. Lightdale, MD
Department of Medicine
Division of Digestive and Liver Diseases
Columbia University Medical Center
161 Fort Washington Avenue
New York, NY 10032, USA

E-mail address:
CJL18@columbia.edu

Preface

Lumen-Apposing Stents: An Important Step Forward

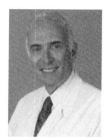

Jacques Van Dam, MD, PhD
Editor

The past two generations of gastroenterologists have witnessed their interventional endoscopist colleagues facilitate diagnostic and therapeutic maneuvers previously in the realm of interventional radiology and general surgery. Connecting two distinct lumens is the basis of many special procedures in gastrointestinal surgery, and for that matter, vascular surgery as well. The ability to bring together and connect two lumens endoscopically represents an important step forward in the evolution of our practice.

The so-called sutureless anastomosis was first conceived and reported nearly 200 years ago by Denan (1826), who proposed promoting local ischemia and subsequent healing at the site of connectivity.[1] John Benjamin Murphy, a name well known to our surgical colleagues, introduced a metal device in 1892 designed to compress the tissue of two adjacent loops of bowel and create local ischemia/healing resulting in a sutureless anastomosis. I was first introduced to "Murphy's button" by Jeffrey Ponsky, MD (who keeps one in a display case in his office!). Nonetheless, as clever as our forefathers were when designing devices to connect gastrointestinal lumens, they could not have conceived of creating an alloy of nickel and titanium (nitinol) and using its unique properties to design an endoscopically deployable stent.

The endoscopic deployment of lumen-apposing metal stents (LAMS) represents a relatively new advance in our practice. While novel technologies sometimes require what often feels like an eternity to gain widespread acceptance, the introduction of LAMS was favored in part because of the endoscopically complicated procedures it replaced (drainage of pancreatic pseudocysts and walled-off necrosis) and the frontiers it has opened (rescue of failed biliary drainage, access to the diseased gallbladder, and so forth).

I am indebted to the authors who in every case are the undisputed leaders in this field for their unselfish willingness to contribute to this issue of *Gastrointestinal Endoscopy*

Gastrointest Endoscopy Clin N Am 28 (2018) xiii–xiv
https://doi.org/10.1016/j.giec.2018.01.001
1052-5157/18/© 2018 Published by Elsevier Inc.

giendo.theclinics.com

Clinics of North America. For the novice, this issue serves as an important guide to the indications and step-by-step methods for deploying LAMS. For the expert, this issue serves as a reminder of the complications sometimes encountered when using LAMS, and importantly, their optimal management. For the skeptic, this issue serves as the rationale for the use of LAMS, the safety and efficacy for current indications, and the potential for the future innovation. And, for the historian, please see Kenneth F. Binmoeller and Andrew Nett's article, "The Evolution of Endoscopic Cystgastrostomy," in this issue for a front-row seat to how we got here. I am sincerely grateful to all of the authors for contributing their valuable time and expertise.

Jacques Van Dam, MD, PhD
Keck School of Medicine
The University of Southern California
1510 San Pablo Street
Suite 322R
Los Angeles, CA 90033, USA

REFERENCE

1. Amat C. Appareils a sutures: les viroles de Denans; les points de Bonnier; Les boutons de Murphy. Arch Med Pharmacie Millitaires Paris 1985;25:273–85.

Fluid Collections and Pseudocysts as a Complication of Acute Pancreatitis

Jack Braha, MD[a], Scott Tenner, MD, MPH[b],*

KEYWORDS

- Pseudocysts • Pancreatic necrosis • Acute pancreatitis • Fluid collections
- Drainage

KEY POINTS

- A pseudocyst may occur secondary to acute pancreatitis, pancreatic trauma, or chronic pancreatitis. Pseudocysts usually contain a high concentration of pancreatic enzymes and variable amounts of tissue debris. Most are sterile.
- In the absence of a clear history of acute pancreatitis or chronic pancreatitis, a pancreatic cystic lesion will rarely be a pseudocyst.
- An acute fluid collection is fluid located in or near the pancreas that lacks a definite wall and typically occurs early in the course of acute pancreatitis.
- It is very difficult to distinguish acute fluid collections in the pancreatic parenchyma from pancreatic necrosis, as well as walled-off pancreatic necrosis from pseudocysts.
- Treatment choices of symptomatic pseudocysts include surgical, radiologic, and endoscopic drainage. No randomized prospective trials have adequately compared these methods.

THE NATURAL HISTORY OF ACUTE PANCREATITIS

Acute pancreatitis is among the most common diseases of the gastrointestinal tract, often leading to significant emotional, physical, and financial human burden. Clinicians often have difficulty managing patients with acute pancreatitis because the disease is complicated by an obscure pathogenesis, few effective remedies, and unpredictable outcome. The incidence of acute pancreatitis seems to be increasing.[1,2] The increase in incidence is most likely related to the relative increasing body mass index and the

Disclosures: The authors have no disclosures.
[a] Division of Gastroenterology, Mount Sinai Medical Center–Brooklyn, The Greater New York Endoscopy Surgical Center, 2211 Emmons Avenue, Brooklyn, NY 11235, USA; [b] State University of New York, The Greater New York Endoscopy Center, 2211 Emmons Avenue, Brooklyn, NY 11235, USA
* Corresponding author.
E-mail address: DrTenner@BrooklynGI.com

Gastrointest Endoscopy Clin N Am 28 (2018) 123–130
https://doi.org/10.1016/j.giec.2017.11.001
1052-5157/18/© 2017 Elsevier Inc. All rights reserved.

increased prevalence of obesity. Because the population is becoming increasingly overweight, the incidence of gallstones, the most common cause of acute pancreatitis is rising. Fortunately, at the same time, the overall mortality rate from acute pancreatitis has gradually declined to approximately 3% to 5%.[3] This is likely due to a better understanding of the pathogenesis and treatment of the disease.[4]

Acute pancreatitis seems to have 2 distinct stages.[5] The first stage is related to the pathophysiology of the inflammatory cascade. This first phase usually lasts a week. During this phase, the severity of acute pancreatitis is related to organ failure secondary to the patient's systemic inflammatory response elicited by acinar cell injury. Fluid extravasates to the peripancreatic regions and is often referred to as acute fluid collections. Infectious complications are uncommon at this time. The fever, tachycardia, hypotension, respiratory distress, and leukocytosis are typically related to the activation of the systemic inflammatory response syndrome. Multiple cytokines are involved, including platelet-activating factor, tumor necrosis factor, and other interleukins.[4]

During the first week, the initial state of inflammation evolves dynamically with variable degrees of pancreatic and peripancreatic ischemia and/or edema, to either resolution or to irreversible necrosis and liquefaction, and/or the development of fluid collections in and around the pancreas. The extent of the pancreatic and peripancreatic changes is usually proportional to the severity of organ failure. However, organ failure may develop independent of pancreatic necrosis.[5]

Approximately 75% to 80% of patients with acute pancreatitis have a resolution of the disease process (interstitial pancreatitis) and do not enter the second phase. However, in one-quarter of patients, a more protracted course develops, typically associated with organ failure, often related to the necrotizing process (necrotizing pancreatitis), lasting weeks to months. The mortality peak in the second phase is related to a combination of factors, including organ failure secondary to sterile necrosis, or infected necrosis or complications from surgical intervention.

Similar to the 2 phases of the disease process, there are 2 peaks for mortality. Most studies in the United States and Europe reveal that about one-half the deaths occur within the first or second week of the disease, usually of multiorgan failure.[6] Death can be very rapid. About one-quarter of all deaths in Scotland occur within 24 hours of admission and one-third within 48 hours.[7] After the second week of illness, patients succumb to pancreatic infection associated with multiorgan failure. Some studies in Europe report a very high rate of late mortality from infection. Patients who are older and have comorbid illnesses have a substantially higher rate of mortality than younger healthier patients. In those who survive their illness, severe pancreatic necrosis can scar the pancreas, resulting in a stricture of the main pancreatic duct with subsequent recurrent attacks of disease, chronic pancreatitis, and/or recurrent pseudocyst formation.

DEFINITIONS

Acute pancreatitis is best defined clinically as the diagnosis for a patient presenting with 2 of the following criteria: (1) symptoms, such as epigastric pain, consistent with the disease; (2) a serum amylase and/or lipase greater than 3 times the upper limit of normal; or (3) radiologic imaging consistent with the diagnosis via computed tomography (CT), and/or MRI.[3] Although the diagnosis of acute pancreatitis is easily determined early in the course of the disease, the severity of the disease requires vigilance because the severity of the disease is not accurately defined for the first 48 hours.[5]

After the diagnosis is established, within 48 hours of the disease, patients are classified as having severe or moderately severe or mild disease.[5] Mild acute pancreatitis consists of minimal or no organ dysfunction, interstitial (edematous) pancreatitis on imaging, and an uneventful recovery. Severe pancreatitis manifests as persistent organ failure. Moderately severe acute pancreatitis is defined as reversible organ failure lasting less than 48 hours and/or local complications such as necrosis, abscess, or pseudocyst. Historically, the presence of pseudocysts defined severe disease; however, in the new Atlanta Guidelines,[5] in the absence of persistent organ failure, the presence of pseudocysts does not define severe disease. See **Table 1**.

ANATOMIC COMPLICATIONS OF ACUTE PANCREATITIS: IMAGING OF PSEUDOCYSTS

It is important to use precise terms in describing the anatomic complications of acute pancreatitis. The ability to apply appropriate therapy depends on a clear understanding of these terms. An old term that should not be used any further is phlegmon. Although this term is often used by radiologists describing an inflammatory mass, this term has carried different meanings to gastroenterologists, internists, radiologists, and surgeons. Whereas patients with interstitial pancreatitis have a normally perfused gland, thus a normal bright appearance indicating flow throughout the gland on contrast-enhanced CT, patients with necrotizing pancreatitis have greater than 30% of the gland not perfused, with low attenuation. Pancreatic necrosis consists of focal or diffuse nonviable pancreatic parenchyma and, usually, peripancreatic fat necrosis.[8]

Unlike pancreatic necrosis, which arises from ischemic pancreatic parenchyma, pseudocysts arise from fluid collections.[9] A pseudocyst may occur secondary to acute pancreatitis, pancreatic trauma, or chronic pancreatitis. It usually contains a high concentration of pancreatic enzymes and variable amounts of tissue debris. Most are sterile. However, a pseudocyst may become infected and then referred to as an abscess. Similar to the treatment of all abscesses, drainage and broad-spectrum antibiotics are typically needed.

Table 1	
Definitions of severity in acute pancreatitis: comparison of Atlanta and recent revision	
Atlanta Criteria (1993)	**Atlanta Revision (2013)**
Mild acute pancreatitis	Mild acute pancreatitis
Absence of organ failure	Absence of organ failure
Absence of local complications	Moderately severe acute pancreatitis
Severe acute pancreatitis (either)	1. Local complications or
Local complications:	pancreatic necrosis
Pancreatic necrosis[a]	Peripancreatic fluid collections
Pseudocysts	Peripancreatic necrosis
Abscess	2. Transient organ failure (<48 h) or
Organ failure	3. Exacerbation of underlying disease
Shock–systolic pressure <90 mm Hg	Severe acute pancreatitis
Pao$_2$ ≤60 mm Hg	Persistent organ failure >48 h
Creatinine >2.0 mg/L after rehydration	
Gastrointestinal bleeding >500 mL/24 h	

[a] Although The Atlanta Symposium defined local complications to include pseudocysts, abscess, and pancreatic necrosis. The interpretation has been that only sterile or infected pancreatic necrosis defines severity as a local complication. Mild acute pancreatitis has no organ failure, local or systemic complications, and usually resolves in the first week. Moderately severe acute pancreatitis is defined by the presence of transient organ failure, local complications, or exacerbation of co-morbid disease. Severe acute pancreatitis is defined by persistent organ failure for more than 48 hours. Local complications are peripancreatic fluid collections, pancreatic and peripancreatic necrosis (sterile or infected), pseudocyst, and walled-off necrosis (sterile or infected).

When approached with the patient with a pseudocyst, the first aspect in care requires verification that the lesion is in fact a pseudocyst, defined as a fluid-filled cystic structure in the pancreas or near the pancreas, rich in pancreatic enzymes, and surrounded by a fibrous wall of tissue. It is important to remember that radiologists often do not have clinical information on the patient and may inappropriately call a fluid collection or any cystic lesion a pseudocyst. In the absence of a clear history of acute pancreatitis or chronic pancreatitis, a pancreatic cystic lesion will rarely be a pseudocyst.

In patients with acute pancreatitis, at least 4 weeks should pass after admission before a fibrous wall forms. Early in the course of acute pancreatitis, calling a fluid collection a pseudocyst is inappropriate. In a patient with no past medical history of chronic pancreatitis, who presents with acute pancreatitis and is found on admission to have a cystic lesion that appears to be a pseudocyst, the lesion may very likely be a cystic neoplasm rather than a pseudocyst.

The treatments of pseudocysts, pancreatic necrosis, and a cystic neoplasm are quite different. Although the absence of a clinical history of acute pancreatitis will help distinguish a pancreatic cystic neoplasm, the differentiation from pancreatic necrosis that becomes walled off; namely, a walled-off pancreatic necrosis (WOPN), from a pseudocyst can be difficult. An acute fluid collection is fluid located in or near the pancreas that lacks a definite wall and typically occurs early in the course of acute pancreatitis. Sometimes, these collections can become infected and may require drainage. After 4 weeks, the fluid collection now has a fibrous wall. On CT scan, these collections are a low-attenuation mass with poor margins and no capsule.[10] It is very difficult to distinguish acute fluid collections in the pancreatic parenchyma from pancreatic necrosis, as well as WOPN from pseudocysts.

A true pseudocyst is a WOPN located adjacent or off the body of the pancreas. At times, these enzyme-rich fluid-filled sacks can be found distantly in the pelvis and chest. When a pseudocyst is located within the body of the pancreas, despite having low attenuation and being fluid-appearing, the cyst may contain necrotic pancreatic debris. The better term for these lesions that are walled-off, fluid-appearing, pseudocyst-like structures involving the pancreas is WOPN. **Figs. 1–3** demonstrate the similar appearance and the way to differentiate between the 2 cystic structures.[11–13]

A pancreatic abscess is a circumscribed intraabdominal collection of pus after an episode of acute pancreatitis or pancreatic trauma. It usually develops close to the pancreas and contains little pancreatic necrosis. Due to confusion of whether an abscess represents an infected pseudocyst or infected pancreatic necrosis, the term

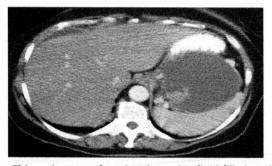

Fig. 1. Pseudocyst. This patient was found to have this fluid-filled, walled-off collection 2 months after an attack of acute pancreatitis. She was unable to tolerate normal meals. After developing postprandial pain and persistent weight loss, endoscopic drainage performed.

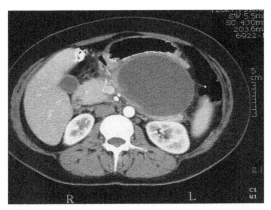

Fig. 2. Pancreatic necrosis. Two weeks after an admission for acute pancreatitis, this patient developed a fever and was found to have this cystic lesion in the pancreas. Although the radiologist wrote that the patient had a pseudocyst, this lesion is pancreatic necrosis. Drainage, if needed, would require surgical intervention due to the solid components in the cyst.

should be used sparingly. Due to important differences in management, it is best to use the terms infected pseudocyst and infected necrosis. Hemorrhagic pancreatitis should not be used as a synonym for necrotizing pancreatitis. The term hemorrhagic pancreatitis should also be used with caution. Hemorrhage is more commonly associated with pseudoaneurysm, an erosion of peripancreatic blood vessels with hemoperitoneum. Unfortunately, the term hemorrhagic pancreatitis has more commonly been used to inappropriately describe necrotizing pancreatitis.

MANAGEMENT OF PSEUDOCYSTS IN ACUTE PANCREATITIS

Historically, the standard of care required intervention in pseudocysts greater than 6 cm or those that were enlarging on serial imaging. Studies by Yeo and colleagues,[9] and Vitas

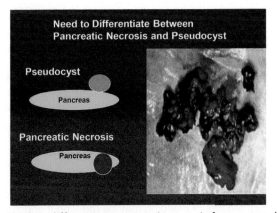

Fig. 3. There is a need to differentiate pancreatic necrosis from a pseudocyst in patients following an attack of acute pancreatitis. On CT imaging, with or without contrast, the cystic lesions have similar Hounsfield units and attenuation is similar. Whereas patients with pseudocysts have the cyst outside the pancreas, patients with pancreatic necrosis have the cyst within the pancreatic parenchyma. Although the cyst appears fluid-filled by CT criteria, the cyst in the pancreatic parenchyma contains debris and often is mostly solid, requiring surgical drainage.

and Sarr,[14] showed that asymptomatic pseudocysts that develop after an attack of acute pancreatitis, regardless of size, can be managed conservatively (ie, no intervention). Current guidelines have built on their data and now recommend that, regardless of size, an asymptomatic pseudocyst does not require treatment.[15] It is satisfactory to monitor the pseudocyst with abdominal ultrasonography every 3 to 6 months.

Pseudocysts can be complicated by infection, intracystic hemorrhage, or rupture leading to pancreatic ascites.[16] Further, pseudocysts can migrate into the chest or other unusual locations. In patients with known pseudocysts, new symptoms, such as abdominal pain, chills, or fever, should alert the clinician to the emergence of an infected pseudocyst or abscess. Pseudocysts can become infected and, when this occurs, they are best described as an abscess (abscesses require drainage). Pseudocysts can become painful, especially in patients with chronic pancreatitis. Pseudocysts can also cause early satiety and weight loss when their size affects the stomach and bowel. When confronted with a patient who has a symptomatic pseudocyst, whether it is infected or painful, drainage is recommended.

Treatment choices include surgical, radiologic, and endoscopic drainage. No randomized prospective trials have compared these methods.[17] Surgical drainage of a pseudocyst is possible with a cystogastrostomy or cystoduodenostomy if the pseudocyst wall is broadly adherent to the stomach or duodenum.[18,19] Other procedures include a Roux-en-Y cystojejunostomy or pancreatic resection if the pseudocyst is in the tail. Surgical mortality is 6% or less. Pseudocyst recurrence after internal drainage occurs in 15% of cases and is more frequent if the main pancreatic duct is obstructed downstream from the surgical anastomosis. For this reason, some experts recommend that a preoperative endoscopic retrograde cholangiopancreatography (ERCP) be usually done to determine whether there is duct obstruction. In this case, a resection of the pseudocyst is preferred.

Percutaneous catheter drainage is an effective treatment to drain and close both sterile and infected pseudocysts. As with surgical drainage, percutaneous catheter drainage may fail if there is obstruction of the main pancreatic duct downstream from the pseudocyst. Therefore, an ERCP is usually done before attempting catheter drainage.

Endoscopic approaches are evolving and becoming increasingly successful.[20,21] Two endoscopic methods to decompress a pancreatic pseudocyst are (1) an endoscopic cystogastrostomy or cystoduodenostomy, or (2) insertion of a stent through the ampulla directly into the pancreatic duct and then into the pseudocyst itself.[22–24] The former method is possible if the pseudocyst is broadly adherent to the wall of the stomach or duodenum. The endoscopist then inserts a double-pigtail stent through the hollow viscus into the cyst. Some endoscopists also insert a transpapillary pancreatic duct stent into the cyst. This is possible if ERCP shows continuity between the pseudocyst and the main pancreatic duct. With either method, the catheter is removed after 3 to 4 weeks if closure of the pseudocyst is seen by CT scan. Failure of radiologic or endoscopic drainage of a pancreatic pseudocyst increases morbidity and prolongs hospitalization. However, most series show long-term resolution with successful endoscopic drainage of pseudocysts.

There are several complications of endoscopic drainage of pseudocysts. The most important is bleeding; the risk of bleeding may be reduced if endoscopic ultrasonography is used to be certain that there are no large vessels in the drainage area. Infection may occur if the double-pigtail catheter becomes occluded. A nasocystic drain to irrigate the cyst may prevent this complication. An endoscopically placed stent in the pancreatic duct may induce ductal changes identical to those of chronic pancreatitis. For this reason, a stent should be removed after several weeks.

If a pseudocyst accompanies considerable pancreatic necrosis, endoscopic and percutaneous catheter drainage should be used very cautiously because neither technique can evacuate the underlying particulate necrotic material, although both are successful in eliminating the fluid of the pseudocyst itself. In this situation, surgical drainage may be preferred because necrotic debris can be retrieved before completing the cystoenteric anastomosis.[25]

SUMMARY

The first aspect in the evaluation of a pseudocyst is determining whether the cyst is truly a pseudocyst. Although medical therapy is not likely to be beneficial in pseudocyst, drainage is beneficial in patients with symptomatic disease. From multiple case series, it seems that pain, early satiety, and infection will be relieved by drainage of the pseudocyst. There are currently no randomized controlled studies comparing the various minimally invasive approaches in the management of pancreatic pseudocysts. Depending on the available local expertise and technology, intervention should be applied. It remains unclear whether an ERCP is necessary to document communication with the main pancreatic duct to attempt a transpapillary approach compared with a transmural approach. Further study will be needed to clarify the best approach to managing pseudocysts complicating chronic pancreatitis. Due to the minimal invasiveness, reported safety, and success rates of the approach in the literature, if expertise is available, an endoscopic approach is preferred.

REFERENCES

1. Peery AE, Dellon ES, Lund J, et al. Burden of gastrointestinal diseases in the United States: 2012 update. Gastroenterology 2012;143:1179–87.
2. Fagenholz PJ, Castillo CF, Harris NS, et al. Increasing United States hospital admissions for acute pancreatitis, 1988-2003. Ann Epidemiol 2007;17:491–7.
3. Yadav D, Lowenfels AB. Trends in the epidemiology of the first attack of acute pancreatitis: a systemic review. Pancreas 2006;33:323–30.
4. Tenner SM. Initial management of acute pancreatitis: critical issues during the first 72 hours. Am J Gastroenterol 2004;99:2489–94.
5. Banks PA, Bollen TL, Dervenis C, et al. Classification of acute pancreatitis – 2012: revision of Atlanta classification and definitions by international consensus. Gut 2013;62(1):102–11.
6. Mofidi R, Duff MD, Wigmore SJ, et al. Association between early systemic inflammatory response, severity of multiorgan dysfunction and death in acute pancreatitis. Br J Surg 2006;93(6):738–44.
7. Buter A, Imrie CW, Carter CR, et al. Dynamic nature of early organ dysfunction determines outcome in acute pancreatitis. Br J Surg 2002;89:298–302.
8. Baril NB, Ralls PW, Wren SM, et al. Does an infected peripancreatic fluid collection or abscess mandate operation? Ann Surg 2000;231:361–7.
9. Yeo CJ, Bastidas JA, Lynch-Nyhan A, et al. The natural history of pancreatic pseudocysts documented by computed tomography. Surg Gynecol Obstet 1990;170:411.
10. Beger HG, Rau B, Isenmann R. Natural history of necrotizing pancreatitis. Pancreatology 2003;3:93–101.
11. Siddiqui AA, Adler DG, Nieto J, et al. EUS-guided drainage of peripancreatic fluid collections and necrosis by using a novel lumen-apposing stent: a large retrospective, multicenter U.S. experience (with videos). Gastrointest Endosc 2016; 83:699–707.

12. Busquets J, Fabregat J, Pelaez N, et al. Factors influencing mortality in patients undergoing surgery for acute pancreatitis: importance of peripancreatic tissue and fluid infection. Pancreas 2013;42(2):285–92.
13. Baron TH, Harewood GC, Morgan DE, et al. Outcome differences after endoscopic drainage of pancreatic necrosis, acute pancreatic pseudocysts, and chronic pancreatic pseudocysts. Gastrointest Endosc 2002;56:7–17.
14. Vitas GJ, Sarr MG. Selected management of pancreatic pseudocysts: operative versus expectant management. Surgery 1992;111:123.
15. Tenner S, Vege S, DeWitt J, et al. Acute pancreatitis: guidelines for the American College of Gastroenterology. Am J Gastroenterol 2013;108(9):1400–15.
16. Flati G, Andren-Sandberg A, La Pinta M, et al. Potentially fatal bleeding in acute pancreatitis: pathophysiology, prevention and treatment. Pancreas 2003;26:8–14.
17. Selvan K, Gurusamy E, Pallari N, et al. Management strategies for pancreatic pseudocysts. Cochrane Database Syst Rev 2016;(4):CD011392.
18. Zhou ZG, Zheng YC, Shu Y, et al. Laparoscopic management of severe acute pancreatitis. Pancreas 2003;27:46–50.
19. Holt BA, Varadarajulu S. The endoscopic management of pancreatic pseudocysts (with videos). Gastrointest Endosc 2015;4:804–12.
20. Lawson JM, Baillie J. Endoscopic therapy for pancreatic pseudocysts. Gastrointest Endosc Clin N Am 1995;5:181.
21. Catalano MF, Geenen JE, Schmalz MJ, et al. Treatment of pancreatic pseudocysts with ductal communication by transpapillary pancreatic duct endoprosthesis. Gastrointest Endosc 1995;42:214.
22. Walter D, Will U, Sanchez-Yague A, et al. A novel lumen-apposing metal stent for endoscopic ultrasound-guided drainage of pancreatic fluid collections: A prospective cohort study. Endoscopy 2015;47:63–7.
23. Shah RJ, Shah JN, Waxman I, et al. Safety and efficacy of endoscopic ultrasound-guided drainage of pancreatic fluid collections with lumen-apposing covered self-expanding metal stents. Clin Gastroenterol Hepatol 2015;13:747–52.
24. Lee BU, Song TJ, Lee SS, et al. Newly designed, fully covered metal stents for endoscopic ultrasound (EUS)-guided transmural drainage of peripancreatic fluid collections: a prospective randomized study. Endoscopy 2014;46:1078–84.
25. Cotton PB, Eisen GM, Aabakken L, et al. A lexicon for endoscopic adverse events: report of an ASGE workshop. Gastrointest Endosc 2010;71:450–4.

Surgical Management of Pancreatic Pseudocysts

Lea Matsuoka, MD*, Sophoclis P. Alexopoulos, MD

KEYWORDS

- Pancreatic pseudocysts • Cystogastrostomy • Laparoscopy • Pancreatitis

KEY POINTS

- Open surgical intervention for pancreatic pseudocysts has a high success rate but significant morbidity.
- Laparoscopic surgical techniques for pancreatic pseudocysts are safe and feasible with possible improvements in complications and length of stay.
- Surgical treatment of pseudocysts in the setting of chronic pancreatitis should treat the underlying parenchymal and ductal disease.
- Multidisciplinary team effort is necessary for the successful treatment of pancreatic pseudocysts.

Pancreatic pseudocysts (PPs) develop in 40% of patients with chronic pancreatitis and 15% of patients with acute pancreatitis.[1] These pseudocysts are persistent peripancreatic fluid collections with a well-defined wall. Indications for intervention include infection, rupture, bleeding, or obstruction of adjacent structures, which can lead to symptoms, such as bloating, nausea and vomiting, abdominal pain, and jaundice. Open surgical intervention was previously the gold standard for treatment of PP with its inherent risk of morbidity and mortality. The advent of minimally invasive techniques, however, has led to an increase in available treatment options.

The treatment approach to PP should be individualized and take multiple factors into consideration. These multiple factors include underlying acute versus chronic pancreatitis; the development of symptoms caused by the PP or complications, such as venous thrombosis or biliary obstruction, the location of the pseudocyst, and single versus multiple PPs and the status of the pancreatic duct.[2–4] Surgical management of uncomplicated PPs in the setting of acute pancreatitis, PPs and chronic pancreatitis, and complicated PPs are discussed separately.

The authors have no disclosures.
Department of Surgery, Vanderbilt University, 801 Oxford House, 1313 21st Avenue South, Nashville, TN 37232, USA
* Corresponding author.
E-mail address: lea.matsuoka@vanderbilt.edu

Gastrointest Endoscopy Clin N Am 28 (2018) 131–141
https://doi.org/10.1016/j.giec.2017.11.002
1052-5157/18/© 2017 Elsevier Inc. All rights reserved.

giendo.theclinics.com

UNCOMPLICATED PANCREATIC PSEUDOCYSTS AFTER ACUTE PANCREATITIS

Uncomplicated PPs that develop after an episode of acute pancreatitis are persistent, simple fluid collections with no necrosis or debris that have a mature wall and can become symptomatic. A majority of published studies include this group of patients with uncomplicated retrogastric PPs. These patients usually have otherwise normal pancreatic parenchyma and normal pancreatic ducts. In 2002, Nealon and Walser[2] correlated the success of PP drainage with pancreatic ductal anatomy and emphasized the importance of the pancreatic ductal anatomy in determining appropriate treatment of PP. Patients with uncomplicated PP are candidates for successful internal drainage procedures as treatment of their symptomatic PP. Correspondingly, PPs in the head, uncinate process, neck, and body of the pancreas may also be amenable to transpapillary endoscopic drainage if there is communication between the PP and the pancreatic duct. PPs located in the tail of the pancreas or in areas distant from the pancreas do not usually respond to transpapillary endoscopic drainage and, therefore, should be considered for internal drainage or resection.

Once a decision has been made to perform internal drainage for the treatment of a PP, the next branch point in the decision tree is whether to approach the drainage with surgery or endoscopy. A majority of PPs are located posterior to the stomach and abuts the stomach or duodenum, making them amenable to both surgical and endoscopic intervention (**Fig. 1**). The traditional open surgical approach is performed via a midline or bilateral subcostal incision with wide exposure of the stomach and duodenum. In the 1970s and 1980s, success rates were high but postoperative morbidity after surgical intervention for PPs was 30%.[5] In the hopes of decreasing operative morbidity and mortality associated with an open approach, the first descriptions of laparoscopic internal drainage of PPs were reported in 1994.[6] Multiple publications since that time have demonstrated the efficacy and feasibility of the laparoscopic approach.[7–10] Typically, patients are placed in the supine position and 3 port sites are used. The surgeon may be on the right side of the patient or between the patient's legs. The camera port is placed in the supraumbilical midline with 2 working ports in the left and right midclavicular lines. On entering the abdomen, the retrogastric PP

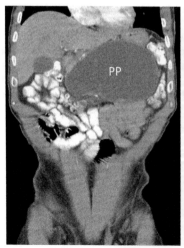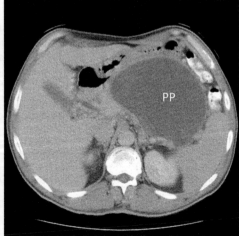

Fig. 1. CT images demonstrating uncomplicated retrogastric pancreatic pseudocyst, amenable to surgical or endoscopic intervention.

often can be seen causing bulging of the stomach (**Fig. 2**). The PP is approached in an anterior fashion through the anterior wall of the stomach, which is opened using harmonic scalpel or electrocautery (**Fig. 3**). Aspiration or ultrasound may be used to confirm the position of the PP. Drainage is achieved by performing a cystogastrostomy at least 4 cm to 5 cm long between the posterior wall of the stomach and the anterior wall of the PP using a laparoscopic stapler or electrocautery. One of the advantages of the laparoscopic surgical approach is the ability to create a large stoma and control any bleeding from the stomach wall. The PP is drained and any necessary pancreatic débridement can be performed, which is another advantage of a surgical approach (**Fig. 4**). The walls of the cystogastrostomy can then be oversewn to prevent bleeding or narrowing of the stoma. The anterior wall of the stomach is closed with stapler or running suture (**Fig. 5**). An alternative posterior approach may be used by entering the lesser sac and creating a cystogastrostomy between the posterior wall of the stomach and the anterior wall of the cyst and then closing or oversewing the cystogastrostomy. PPs that are not retrogastric are amenable to open or laparoscopic approaches. **Fig. 6** shows a pelvic PP that was treated with Roux-en-Y cystojejunostomy (see **Fig. 6**).

Park and Heniford[8] in 2002 published the largest series at that time of 29 patients undergoing laparoscopic PP surgery. They described a transgastric anterior approach, posterior lesser sac approach, and cystojejunostomy. The investigators concluded that although the series was small with short-term follow-up, laparoscopic techniques for treatment of PP were feasible. Subsequently, Palanivelu and colleagues[9] reported on 90 patients from a single center who underwent laparoscopic cystogastrostomy and 8 patients who underwent laparoscopic cystojejunostomy. The laparoscopic cystogastrostomies were all performed using an anterior transgastric approach. With a mean follow-up time of 54 months, there were no mortalities, no conversions to open procedure, and only 1 recurrence. In the first case-matched comparative study published, Khaled and colleagues[11] performed a comparison between 30 patients who underwent laparoscopic cystogastrostomy compared with 10 matched patients who underwent open cystogastrostomy. The laparoscopic group had statistically shorter operative times (62 min vs 95 min), decreased complication rates (10% vs 60%), and shorter length of stay (6.2 days vs 11 days) compared with the open group. Follow-up for these patients was 1 year. Although the vast majority of literature

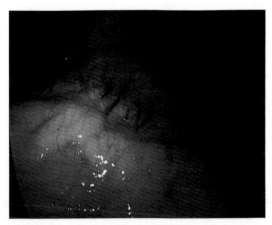

Fig. 2. Intraoperative laparoscopic view of a retrogastric pancreatic pseudocyst anteriorly displacing the stomach.

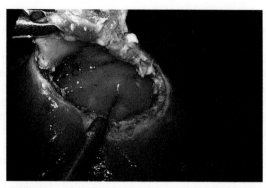

Fig. 3. Intraoperative laparoscopic view of a retrogastric pancreatic pseudocyst. The anterior wall of the stomach has been open and a needle is inserted into the posterior wall of the stomach into the retrogastric pancreatic pseudocyst.

regarding laparoscopic PP surgery continues to be case reports and case series, laparoscopic techniques seem feasible with the potential for advantages over the open approach in terms of complications and length of stay.

The bigger area of controversy remains in the area of operative intervention versus endoscopic approaches. In 2007, Aljarabah and Ammori[12] performed a systematic review of cohort series looking at the laparoscopic and endoscopic treatment of PPs. At that time, there were no published randomized or comparative studies; 19 cohort series on the laparoscopic approach and 25 cohort series on the endoscopic approach were reviewed, which included 118 laparoscopic and 569 endoscopic patients. The laparoscopic approach compared with endoscopic approach success rate was 98% versus 80%, morbidity was 4% versus 12%, mortality was 0% versus 0.4%, and recurrence rate was 2.5% versus 14.4%. The investigators were unable, however, to perform a direct statistical comparison because of heterogeneity of the reports. Although a direct comparison was not possible, these results do demonstrate the relative success and safety of both approaches. In 2008, Melman and colleagues[13] published a retrospective, comparative study among laparoscopic, endoscopic, and open cystogastrostomies for treatment of PPs. The study included 16 laparoscopic, 22 open, and 45 endoscopic patients and reported no difference in complication rates

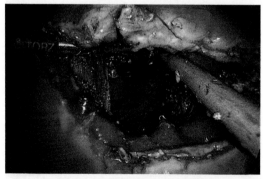

Fig. 4. Intraoperative laparoscopic view of a retrogastric pancreatic pseudocyst. The anterior wall of the stomach has been opened and a stoma created between the posterior wall of the stomach/anterior wall of the pseudocyst. The suction instrument is in the pancreatic pseudocyst cavity, which can be drained and débrided in necessary.

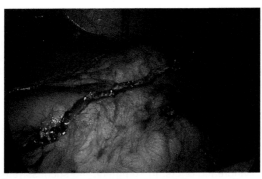

Fig. 5. Intraoperative laparoscopic view of a retrogastric pancreatic pseudocyst. After the creation of a cystogastrostomy and drainage of the pancreatic pseudocyst, the anterior wall of the stomach is stapled or sewn closed.

(31.5% vs 22.7% vs 15.6%, respectively), but there was a higher primary success rate with surgical approach compared with endoscopy (87.5% vs 81.2% vs 51.1%, respectively). When looking at the overall success rate, there was no significant difference noted (92.8% vs 90.9% vs 84.6%, respectively). Of the 45 patients who underwent initial treatment with endoscopy, however, 6 required an additional endoscopy and 13 required an open surgical procedure. In 2009, Johnson and colleagues[14] compared 30 patients who underwent surgical treatment of PP and 24 patients who underwent endoscopy. The details of the surgical interventions (laparoscopic vs open) were not detailed in the study, but 15 surgical patients also underwent additional pancreaticobiliary surgeries, including procedures such as cholecystectomy, splenectomy, and pancreaticojejunostomy. The group reported no difference in complication rates (20% vs 21%) or rates of cyst resolution (93% vs 88%) between the surgical and endoscopic groups.

The only single-center randomized trial in the literature was published by Varadarajulu and colleagues[15] in 2013 at the University of Alabama. The study examined 20 patients who underwent endoscopic cystogastrostomy and 20 patients who

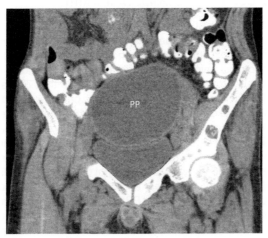

Fig. 6. CT image of pancreatic pseudocyst located in the pelvis. A pseudocyst in this location would be amenable to surgical enteric drainage for treatment.

underwent surgical cystogastrostomy. The endoscopic cystogastrostomy was performed using endoscopic ultrasound with dilation to 15 mm and placement of 2 stents. An endoscopic retrograde cholangiopancreatography (ERCP) was performed at the same time and a pancreatic duct stent was placed if there was evidence of a pancreatic duct leak. The surgeries were performed through an open, midline incision by a single surgeon. When comparing the 2 groups the investigators found no difference in success rates or complications. The length of stay, however, was statistically shorter in the endoscopic group (2 vs 6 days) with lower mean costs. When examining the endoscopic group closely, 10 patients had pancreatic duct stents placed and all underwent repeat pancreatograms. Additionally, 1 patient required 2 ERCP stent procedures. The transgastric stents were removed in 15 patients and remain in 5 patients with disconnected pancreatic ducts. In summary, the success rates were the same between the 2 groups, but the shorter length of stay (and corresponding lower costs) seem to be only with the index admission.

Patients with uncomplicated PP after acute pancreatitis can be treated with endovascular or surgical approaches. The surgical approach has a high success rate and has been the gold standard, but confers the risk of general anesthesia and can be challenging in patients with multiple abdominal surgeries. The laparoscopic surgical approach does not negate the risk of general anesthesia but is feasible and safe and may possibly decrease length of stay and costs for the patient. With the surgical approach, additional procedures, such as cholecystectomy, may be performed in the same setting, and there is the ability to perform necrosectomy if needed. The endoscopic approach has the appeal of potentially shorter hospitalization length of stays and does not require general anesthesia. Although large comparative and randomized studies are lacking, the literature suggests complication rates and rates of recurrence to be similar. There has been a shift in the treatment of PP from surgery to endoscopic approaches.[16] It seems, however, that the trade-off is the potential need for multiple procedures in patients undergoing endoscopic cystogastrostomy. Surgery will always be necessary for rescue procedures after complications from endoscopy and the importance of a multidisciplinary approach to the management of patients with PP cannot be emphasized enough.

PANCREATIC PSEUDOCYSTS AND CHRONIC PANCREATITIS

PPs that arise in the setting of chronic pancreatitis warrant separate consideration, because patients with chronic pancreatitis often have abnormal pancreatic parenchymal disease and multiple strictures throughout the pancreatic duct. The most common symptom, abdominal pain, may be attributed to the PP and/or to the underlying chronic pancreatitis. Usatoff and colleagues[17] described their operative approach in 112 patients with chronic pancreatitis and PP: 56 patients underwent resections, the majority of which were distal pancreatectomies; 48 patients underwent cystojejunostomy; and 18 of these patients additionally had a lateral pancreaticojejunostomy (LPJ) performed if their pancreatic duct was dilated. The reported morbidity rate was 28% with a 3% recurrence rate and a 74% rate of postoperative pain relief. The goal of the surgical procedures was to treat not only the PP but also the underlying chronic pancreatitis. Similarly, Schlosser and colleagues[18] retrospectively described 206 patients with chronic pancreatitis and PP in the head of the pancreas. The majority of these patients had abdominal pain; 169 of these patients also had enlarged pancreatic heads and underwent duodenum-preserving pancreatic head resections (17 patients also had additional ductal drainage procedures performed) and 37 patients underwent Roux-en-Y cystojejunostomy. Median follow-up for both groups was over 6 years. The patients who underwent pancreatic head resection had a statistically higher rate of complete pain relief and the groups had similar rates of complications and mortality. Both of these studies demonstrate the efficacy of treating the underlying chronic pancreatitis in addition to the PP, either with additional resection of the pancreas if there was evidence of localized disease or drainage of a dilated pancreatic duct.

Nealon and Walser[19] described 103 patients with chronic pancreatitis, PP, and a dilated pancreatic duct, 56 of whom underwent LPJ and internal drainage of PP and 47 of whom underwent LPJ alone. All these patients were on narcotics for abdominal pain. The investigators found similar outcomes with regard to length of stay, complication, and mortality rates. Impressively, 87% of patients in the LPJ and drainage of PP group and 89% of patients in the LPD group experienced pain relief and were narcotic-free postoperatively. The mean follow-up for the study was 73 months.

In patients with chronic pancreatitis and PP, consideration should be given not only to drainage of the PP but also to treatment of the underlying disease. Pancreatic ductal drainage procedures in the setting of dilated PD and resection procedures need to be considered.

COMPLICATED PANCREATIC PSEUDOCYSTS

Although the underlying principle in the treatment of PP remains the re-establishment of enteric drainage either through surgical, endoscopic, or transpapillary means, there remain certain situations in which such an approach is ill advised. The intense inflammation associated with the development of a PP can result in erosion or thrombosis of adjacent vasculature. Such situations frequently require resection of the PP and associated pancreas once a patient has been stabilized.

PPs can frequently abut and displace the arterial vasculature. When PP causes external compression on an arterial vessel, however, the high pressure and flow of arterial blood and the structure of arteries, including a tunica media, give the arterial system resilience to thrombosis. The same enzymatic processes, however, associated with the formation of the PP can result in digestion of the arterial wall, resulting in pseudoaneurysm formation and subsequent acute arterial hemorrhage. This process is well described in the literature and may result in frank intraperitoneal hemorrhage or intracystic hemorrhage with or without rupture of the pseudocyst into the peritoneal cavity.[20,21] The most frequent site of arterial hemorrhage is from the splenic artery followed by the gastroduodenal or pancreaticoduodenal arteries.[22] Such hemorrhage is life threatening and must be controlled with stabilization of the patient prior to any definitive therapy for the PP. If available, interventional radiologic (IR) treatment of arterial hemorrhage should be the preferred approach, with surgical control reserved for cases in which IR is unavailable or for patients too unstable for IR therapy. High complication and mortality rates are associated with initial surgical management.[23,24] After control of hemorrhage, definitive treatment of the PP frequently requires surgical resection as opposed to enteric drainage.[25] To mitigate the risk of bleeding complications, PP-threatening erosion into the splenic artery can be successfully treated with distal pancreatectomy and splenectomy, whereas those involving the gastroduodenal or pancreaticoduodenal artery frequently require pancreaticoduodenectomy.

In contrast to the arterial vasculature, the splanchnic venous drainage is a low-pressure, low-flow system uniquely predisposed to thrombosis when compressed by an inflammatory mass. As such, PPs resulting from pancreatitis tend to be associated with thrombosis rather than erosion into the splenic, portal, or superior

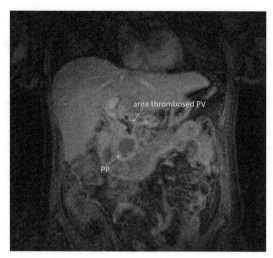

Fig. 7. MRI image showing pancreatic pseudocyst arising from the head/uncinate process of the pancreas, causing thrombosis of the portal vein (PV).

mesenteric veins as they enlarge.[26] Thrombosis of the splenic vein can lead to left-sided portal hypertension with the formation of perigastric varices along the greater curvature of the stomach.[27] These PPs, however, are frequently located in the lesser sac and abutting the stomach and can be successfully treated endoscopically. Although gastric varices were traditionally considered a contraindication to endoscopic treatment, the use of endoscopic ultrasound to guide the posterior gastrostomy and advancements in stent technology have overcome this challenge.[28] PPs arising from the head of the pancreas or growing into the hepatic hilum represent a more significant challenge and are more frequently associated with thrombosis of the portal and/or superior mesenteric vein as well as bile duct obstruction (**Figs. 7** and **8**). Enlarging PPs associated with portal or superior mesenteric vein thrombosis must be treated prior to fistulization of the cyst into the portal venous system.[29] A rare complication of fistulization into the portal venous system is systemic lipolysis,

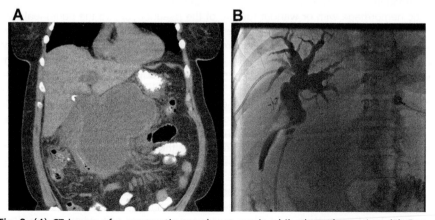

Fig. 8. (A) CT image of a pancreatic pseudocyst causing bile duct obstruction. (B) Corresponding cholangiogram showing bile duct dilation caused by external compression by the pancreatic pseudocyst.

in which pancreatic enzymes enter this systemic circulation, resulting in arthralgias and purpuric subcutaneous nodules representing subcutaneous fat lipolysis.[30,31] Additionally, fistulization becomes a contraindication to enteric drainage of a pseudocyst and an indication for surgical resection of the PP and associated pancreas with repair of the vascular fistula. Closure of the fistula has also been reported with pancreatic duct stenting.[32] Enteric drainage of the PP without closure of the cyst-venous fistula risks recanalization of the venous system with subsequent life-threatening splanchnic hemorrhage into the cyst and intestine.[29]

Although the incidence of significant vascular complications associated with PP is on the decline due to improved imaging, allowing earlier diagnosis and aggressive and effective endoscopic treatments, there remains a small but important role for the surgical treatment and resection of PPs associated with vascular involvement or major vascular hemorrhage or thrombosis.

SUMMARY

The management of PPs requires an individualized, multidisciplinary approach. Patients with symptomatic, uncomplicated PPs located in the retrogastric area and normal pancreatic ducts are candidates for endoscopic or surgical internal drainage procedures. PPs in the head, uncinate process, neck, and body of the pancreas may also be amenable to transpapillary endoscopic drainage if there is communication between the PP and the pancreatic duct. PPs located in the tail of the pancreas or in areas distant from the pancreas should be considered for surgical internal drainage or resection. Laparoscopic surgical approaches have been shown feasible and effective. Patients with chronic pancreatitis and PPs require evaluation of the underlying parenchyma and pancreatic duct. Ductal drainage procedures or resections should be considered. Complicated PPs involving nearby arteries or veins may lead to life-threatening hemorrhage or thrombosis. These situations may require pancreatic resection to prevent or treat these dangerous complications.

REFERENCES

1. Behrns KE, Ben-David K. Surgical therapy of pancreatic pseudocysts. J Gastrointest Surg 2008;12(12):2231–9.
2. Nealon WH, Walser E. Main pancreatic ductal anatomy can direct choice of modality for treating pancreatic pseudocysts (surgery versus percutaneous drainage). Ann Surg 2002;235(6):751–8.
3. Pan G, Wan MH, Xie KL, et al. Classification and management of pancreatic pseudocysts. Medicine (Baltimore) 2015;94(24):e960.
4. Rosso E, Alexakis N, Ghaneh P, et al. Pancreatic pseudocyst in chronic pancreatitis: endoscopic and surgical treatment. Dig Surg 2003;20(5):397–406.
5. Nealon WH, Walser E. Surgical management of complications associated with percutaneous and/or endoscopic management of pseudocyst of the pancreas. Ann Surg 2005;241(6):948–57 [discussion: 957–60].
6. Way L. Laparoscopic pancreatic cystogastrostomy: the first operation in the new field of intraluminal laparoscopic surgery. Surg Endosc 1994;8:235.
7. Beuran M, Negoi I, Catena F, et al. Laparoscopic transgastric versus endoscopic drainage of a large pancreatic pseudocyst. A case report. J Gastrointestin Liver Dis 2016;25(2):243–7.
8. Park AE, Heniford BT. Therapeutic laparoscopy of the pancreas. Ann Surg 2002; 236(2):149–58.

9. Palanivelu C, Senthilkumar K, Madhankumar MV, et al. Management of pancreatic pseudocyst in the era of laparoscopic surgery–experience from a tertiary centre. Surg Endosc 2007;21(12):2262–7.

10. Hamza N, Ammori BJ. Laparoscopic drainage of pancreatic pseudocysts: a methodological approach. J Gastrointest Surg 2010;14(1):148–55.

11. Khaled YS, Malde DJ, Packer J, et al. Laparoscopic versus open cystgastrostomy for pancreatic pseudocysts: a case-matched comparative study. J Hepatobiliary Pancreat Sci 2014;21(11):818–23.

12. Aljarabah M, Ammori BJ. Laparoscopic and endoscopic approaches for drainage of pancreatic pseudocysts: a systematic review of published series. Surg Endosc 2007;21(11):1936–44.

13. Melman L, Azar R, Beddow K, et al. Primary and overall success rates for clinical outcomes after laparoscopic, endoscopic, and open pancreatic cystgastrostomy for pancreatic pseudocysts. Surg Endosc 2009;23(2):267–71.

14. Johnson MD, Walsh RM, Henderson JM, et al. Surgical versus nonsurgical management of pancreatic pseudocysts. J Clin Gastroenterol 2009;43(6):586–90.

15. Varadarajulu S, Bang JY, Sutton BS, et al. Equal efficacy of endoscopic and surgical cystogastrostomy for pancreatic pseudocyst drainage in a randomized trial. Gastroenterology 2013;145(3):583–90.e1.

16. Varadarajulu S, Wilcox CM, Latif S, et al. Management of pancreatic fluid collections: a changing of the guard from surgery to endoscopy. Am Surg 2011;77(12):1650–5.

17. Usatoff V, Brancatisano R, Williamson RC. Operative treatment of pseudocysts in patients with chronic pancreatitis. Br J Surg 2000;87(11):1494–9.

18. Schlosser W, Siech M, Beger HG. Pseudocyst treatment in chronic pancreatitis–surgical treatment of the underlying disease increases the long-term success. Dig Surg 2005;22(5):340–5.

19. Nealon WH, Walser E. Duct drainage alone is sufficient in the operative management of pancreatic pseudocyst in patients with chronic pancreatitis. Ann Surg 2003;237(5):614–20 [discussion: 620–2].

20. Dardik I, Dardik H. Patterns of hemorrhage into pancreatic pseudocysts. Am J Surg 1968;115(6):774–6.

21. Bucknam CA. Arterial hemorrhage in pseudocyst of pancreas. Arch Surg 1966;92(3):405–6.

22. Stabile BE, Wilson SE, Debas HT. Reduced mortality from bleeding pseudocysts and pseudoaneurysms caused by pancreatitis. Arch Surg 1983;118(1):45–51.

23. Carr JA, Cho JS, Shepard AD, et al. Visceral pseudoaneurysms due to pancreatic pseudocysts: rare but lethal complications of pancreatitis. J Vasc Surg 2000;32(4):722–30.

24. Chiu HH, Chen CM, Wang KC, et al. Pancreatic pseudocyst bleeding associated with massive intraperitoneal hemorrhage. Am J Surg 2006;192(1):87–8.

25. Bender JS, Bouwman DL, Levison MA, et al. Pseudocysts and pseudoaneurysms: surgical strategy. Pancreas 1995;10(2):143–7.

26. Harris S, Nadkarni NA, Naina HV, et al. Splanchnic vein thrombosis in acute pancreatitis: a single-center experience. Pancreas 2013;42(8):1251–4.

27. Heider TR, Azeem S, Galanko JA, et al. The natural history of pancreatitis-induced splenic vein thrombosis. Ann Surg 2004;239(6):876–80 [discussion: 880–2].

28. Singhal S, Rotman SR, Gaidhane M, et al. Pancreatic fluid collection drainage by endoscopic ultrasound: an update. Clin Endosc 2013;46(5):506–14.

29. Ng TS, Rochefort H, Czaplicki C, et al. Massive pancreatic pseudocyst with portal vein fistula: case report and proposed treatment algorithm. Pancreatology 2015; 15(1):88–93.
30. Zeller M, Hetz HH. Rupture of a pancreatic cyst into the portal vein. Report of a case of subcutaneous nodular and generalized fat necrosis. JAMA 1966;195(10): 869–71.
31. Hammar AM, Sand J, Lumio J, et al. Pancreatic pseudocystportal vein fistula manifests as residivating oligoarthritis, subcutaneous, bursal and osseal necrosis: a case report and review of literature. Hepatogastroenterology 2002;49(43): 273–8.
32. Noh R, Kim HJ. A pancreatic pseudocyst-portal vein fistula closed by endoscopic pancreatic stent insertion. Gastrointest Endosc 2010;72(5):1103–5.

The Evolution of Endoscopic Cystgastrostomy

Kenneth F. Binmoeller, MD*, Andrew Nett, MD

KEYWORDS

- Endoscopic cystgastrostomy • Pancreatic fluid collection • Walled-off necrosis
- Lumen-apposing metal stents • LAMS

KEY POINTS

- The lumen-apposing metal stent is the first stent specifically designed for endoscopic ultrasound-guided transluminal drainage of extraintestinal fluid collections.
- Together with the "hot" electrocautery-enhanced delivery system, this platform marks the most recent evolutionary stage of endoscopic therapy of pancreatic fluid collections.
- In the last 4 decades, management has progressed from the first attempt at drainage by simple pseudocyst aspiration, to single-device, single maneuver deployment of a lumen-apposing metal stent.
- The lumen-apposing metal stent platform has made endoscopic drainage of pancreatic fluid collections easier and safer, serving as a port for safe entry into the cyst.
- Tools conceived for endoscopic ultrasound-guided transluminal intervention have emerged and are opening the door to new frontiers of endoscopic transluminal therapy.

INTRODUCTION

Historically, pancreatic fluid collection (PFC) drainage has been complex, technically challenging, and time consuming, with one of the highest rates of complications reported for an endoscopic procedure. Over the past decades, we have witnessed a remarkable evolution of endoscopic treatment of PFCs, from simple endoscopic aspiration to endoscopic ultrasound (EUS)-guided drainage using dedicated translumenal devices that enable 1-step access and deployment of a lumen apposing stent (**Fig. 1**). These advances have improved technical and clinical success rates while reducing complications. This article covers the evolutionary milestones.

THE BEGINNING: CYST ASPIRATION

Endoscopic aspiration of a PFC, first described in 1975, represented the first translu-minal application of endoscopic therapy.[1] In this case report, a 31-year-old woman

Disclosures: Dr K.F. Binmoeller is the inventor of the AXIOS stent and delivery system, the NAVIX device, and founder of Xlumena Inc, acquired by Boston Scientific.
Interventional Endoscopy Services, California Pacific Medical Center, 2351 Clay Street, Suite 600, San Francisco, CA 94115, USA
* Corresponding author.
E-mail address: BinmoeK@sutterhealth.org

Gastrointest Endoscopy Clin N Am 28 (2018) 143–156
https://doi.org/10.1016/j.giec.2017.11.003
1052-5157/18/© 2017 Elsevier Inc. All rights reserved.

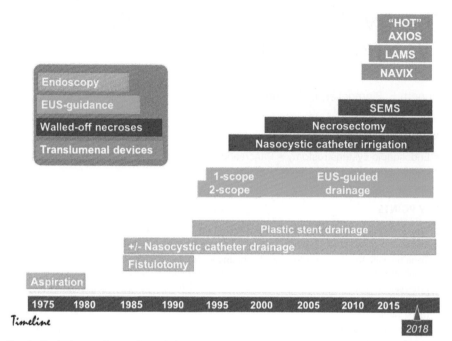

Fig. 1. Evolution and paradigm shifts. EUS, endoscopic ultrasound; LAMS, lumen-apposing metal stent; SEMS, self-expanding metal stents.

diagnosed with a pseudocyst complicating alcoholic pancreatitis had repeated admissions for abdominal pain. An upper gastrointestinal series showed a 10-cm mass with pressure effect onto the stomach, consistent with a pancreatic pseudocyst. Endoscopic aspiration was performed with a 21-G needle that yielded 60 mL of yellow to brown colored, cloudy fluid. The patient had no relief after aspiration, however, and the cyst recurred soon after treatment. Based on the lack of pain relief after endoscopic aspiration, surgical therapy was not pursued, because cyst drainage was thought unlikely to provide symptom relief. Thus, despite the lack of therapeutic benefit, endoscopic cyst aspiration impacted patient management. Of note, expectations for a definitive therapeutic benefit from simple endoscopic aspiration were low in light of prior reports of high recurrence rates after percutaneous cyst aspiration.[2,3]

FISTULOTOMY

In 1985, a decade after the report of ineffective endoscopic cyst aspiration, headway was finally made with the report of pseudocyst drainage via creation of a fistulotomy opening using a diathermic needle knife.[4] Fistulotomy creation was performed using a duodenoscope in 4 high-risk individuals who had either failed surgery or in whom surgery was contraindicated. The fistulotomy incision varied from 0.5 to 1.5 cm. The hypothesis was that, whereas simple needle puncture and aspiration yields temporary and insufficient drainage, the creation of a larger opening more analogous to surgical internal drainage might lead to resolution. PFCs did resolve with endoscopic treatment in 2 patients. Repeat endoscopic fistulotomies were required, however, in 2 of the 4 patients, and in 1 patient a nasocystic catheter was inserted after fistulotomy to gravity drainage as an additional means to obtain drainage. Among the 2 patients with endoscopic failure, 1 patient required surgery and the other expired after treatment without

PFC resolution. Complications consisted of major bleeding in 1 patient that did not require intervention.

NASOCYSTIC CATHETER DRAINAGE

Success of fistulotomy as a sole treatment is limited by the rapid, spontaneous closure of the opening before complete cyst resolution, resulting in cyst recurrence and super-infection. Percutaneous catheter placement, as a method of more prolonged cyst drainage, can achieve high therapeutic success rates, but carries a high risk of pancrea-ticocutaneous fistula formation.[5] Thus, although fistulotomy represented an important advancement in PFC management, the search for an endoscopic solution continued.

To facilitate sustained drainage over time while avoiding external fistulae, prolonged internal cyst drainage by nasocystic catheter drainage was reported in 1987 in a series of 20 patients.[6] A large 10- to 15-mm cystogastrostomy fistulotomy was performed using a needle knife followed by placement of a nasocystic catheter up to 7F in diameter. Irrigation was performed for 1.7 days with isotonic saline. Results were reported as "good" in 47% of patients. There were 2 perforations and 2 bleeds. One bleed was fatal. A second large series of 33 patients treated by nasocystic catheter drainage was reported in 1989 by cystgastrostomy (11 patients) or cystduodenostomy (22 patients).[7] After a 10-mm needle knife fistulotomy, a 6F or 9F nasocystic catheter was inserted and continuous irrigation performed until cyst resolution. Success rates were 100% and 96% for cystgastrostomy and cystduodenostomy, respectively. There were 2 bleeding complications that occurred during fistulotomy and 1 cyst infection that required percutaneous drainage. Patient tolerance of continuous nasocystic catheter drainage was not measured in any of the published studies.

Our experience has been that patients poorly tolerate a nasocystic catheter owing to nasal discomfort and burdensome maintenance. Also, despite best efforts to anchor the catheter with tape to the nose and face, the catheter frequently retracts and pulls out of the cyst. Thus, although it is capable of achieving PFC resolution, endoscopic nasocystic catheter drainage is a suboptimal and impractical solution.

PLASTIC STENT DRAINAGE

Internal stent placement developed as an alternative to nasocystic catheter drainage. The stent acts to maintain patency of the cystgastrostomy or cystduodenostomy fistula while avoiding patient discomfort caused by a nasally routed tube. The off-label use of conventional 7F or 10F plastic biliary stents for transmural PFC drainage was first reported in 2 large series in 1993. Binmoeller and colleagues[8] (Hamburg group) treated 24 patients and Smits and colleagues[9] (Amsterdam group) treated 37 patients for a total of 61 patients. Single stent insertion was performed after a diathermic fistulotomy. Success rates exceeded 90% in both series. Bleeding and perforation, however, occurred in both series (a total of 5 bleeds and 2 perforations). There was 1 inadvertent gallbladder puncture in the Hamburg series.

TWO-SCOPE ENDOSCOPIC ULTRASOUND-GUIDED DRAINAGE

Around the time that plastic stents were applied to PFC therapy, advances in endoso-nographic equipment expanded the role of endoscopic therapy. Using endoscopic visualization alone, only pseudocysts producing a prominent visible bulge into the lumen of the stomach or duodenum were amenable to transmural drainage (**Fig. 2**). The development of the curved linear-array echoendoscope in the early 1990s, which enabled real-time ultrasound visualization of a tool pushed out of the accessory

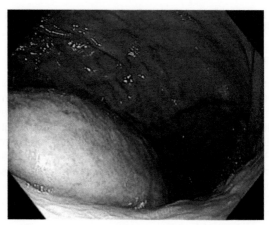

Fig. 2. Extrinsic compression of the stomach by a peripancreatic fluid collection. Such a bulge is required for endoscopic therapy performed without endoscopic ultrasound guidance.

channel, extended the reach of endoscopic drainage to include cysts without an associated bulge in the enteric lumen. In addition, EUS guidance made pseudocyst access theoretically safer, because it enabled the endoscopist to identify and avoid interposed vessels, as well as to identify extraintestinal structures to be avoided during cyst puncture.

EUS-guided pseudocyst drainage using a 2-scope approach was first reported by Binmoeller and the Hamburg group in 1992 in a patient with no visible extrinsic compression ("bulge") on endoscopy.[10] Cyst puncture was performed with a needle knife catheter that allowed the removal of the inner needle followed by insertion of a guidewire through the catheter into the pseudocyst. After guidewire placement, the small working channel (2.0 mm) of this first-generation curved linear-array echoendoscope necessitated scope exchange for a duodenoscope with a large 4.2-mm channel to then insert a 10F plastic stent.

ONE-SCOPE ENDOSCOPIC ULTRASOUND-GUIDED PSEUDOCYST DRAINAGE

The development of larger channel echoendoscopes made stent insertion under EUS guidance possible with a single scope, eliminating the need to exchange the echoendoscope for a larger channel endoscope such as a 4.2-mm channel duodenoscope. Single-scope EUS-guided pseudocyst drainage with a 7F stent inserted through a 2.4-mm echoendoscope was reported in 1996.[11] Subsequent development of 3.7-mm and 3.8-mm working-channel echoendoscopes enabled the placement of a 10F stent.[12]

MULTIPLE PLASTIC STENTS

Endoscopic PFC drainage was further modified over time with development of multistenting techniques in an effort to enhance drainage and minimize complications from stent occlusion. It was postulated that the placement of multiple stents enabled drainage both alongside as well as through the stents. Multistenting became common practice, despite the lack of studies documenting the superiority of 2 or more plastic stents over a single stent for pseudocyst drainage.[13] Even if superior, reinterventions for stent exchange were reported necessary in 17.7% to 27.0% of cases where multiple stents were used.[14,15] The downside of placing multiple plastic stents is a significant increase in procedure time, mainly owing to technically challenges associated with placing the second or third stent alongside the previously inserted device. Several developments over time sought to improve the process of introducing multiple plastic stents by first placing the guidewires through a large bore catheter such as a 10F stent pusher catheter before the insertion of the stents. However, multiple guidewires occupying the working channel compromised the size of plastic stent that could be inserted; as a rule, the first stent inserted alongside 1 or 2 guidewires could not be larger than 7F.

THE SELDINGER TECHNIQUE

Historically, cyst drainage has required multiple coaxial over-the-wire exchanges of various catheter instruments according to the Seldinger technique. After the cyst is accessed under EUS guidance with a 19-G fine needle aspiration needle, a guidewire is inserted and coiled within the cyst. The needle is removed over the wire and exchanged for a dilating instrument (bougie and/or balloon catheter) to prime the transmural tract for stent insertion. Dilation to 6 or 8 mm is typically needed. If necrosectomy is indicated, the tract may be further dilated, usually to 15 or 18 mm, to allow passage of a gastroscope into the cavity. After tract dilation, multiple plastic stents are placed over guidewires. As mentioned, various off-the-shelf, large bore (at least 10F) catheters have been used to enable the simultaneous placement of multiple guidewires followed by sequentially inserted plastic stents. Throughout this entire process, each procedural step risks leakage, perforation, and bleeding, especially when the cyst and bowel walls are not adherent.

PLATFORMS TO COMBINE ACCESS AND TRACT DILATION

Several device platforms have been developed to combine procedural steps of access, dilation, and drainage. The Cystotome (Cook Endoscopy, Winston-Salem, NC) is a double-layered system that consists of an inner, 5F retractable needle-knife catheter and an outer 10F sheath with a metal electrocautery ring at the distal tip. The inner needle-knife is used to diathermically puncture the PFC, after which the outer sheath with the metal tip is coaxially advanced over the inner catheter while applying diathermy current to create a 10F cystenterostomy. The needle-knife catheter is withdrawn, leaving the outer sheath in place within the cyst, and 1 or 2 guidewires are inserted for balloon dilation and/or stent drainage.[16] A prototype "transluminal balloon accessotome" for endoscopy-guided pseudocyst drainage has also been developed, combining needle-knife puncture and balloon dilation in a single step.[17]

The NAVIX device, designed by Binmoeller, enables cyst access, tract dilation, and placement of 2 guidewires with a single device (**Fig. 3**).[18] The device consists of a lumen-less trocar made of nitinol, a switchblade at the trocar tip, an anchor balloon that maintains access within the target, a dilation balloon, and 2 guidewire ports (**Fig. 3A**). Radiopaque and endoscopic markers on the shaft indicate the location of the proximal and distal ends of the balloon, and the location of the second guidewire exit port (**Fig. 3B**). The device handle Luer locks onto the inlet port of the working channel of a curved linear array echoendoscope. The solid 19G trocar provides a stable platform for coaxial advancement of the balloon catheter. The switchblade, flush with the trocar when constrained by the catheter sheath, deploys to a 45° angle upon retraction of the catheter sheath. The switchblade creates a 3.5-mm puncture opening in the wall upon advancement across the wall of the cyst. After trocar puncture, the 10F balloon catheter is advanced over the trocar into the cyst. The dilation balloon has a "dog-bone" configuration to stabilize the position across the wall during balloon inflation and counter the tendency for the balloon to slip forward or backward. The distal anchor balloon remains inflated during the entire procedure to prevent

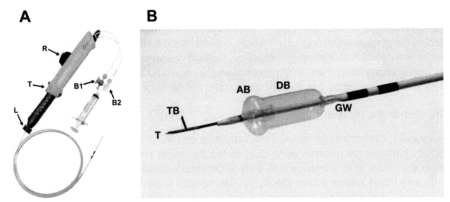

Fig. 3. (*A*) Overview of the NAVIX device. At the handle end, separate ports B1 and B2 are used to inflate the anchor and dilation balloons, respectively. The balloon catheter is advanced using a rotating knob (R). The depth of trocar advancement is set with the trocar depth collar (T). The handle is Luer fitted (L) onto the echoendoscope working channel inlet port. (*B*) The NAVIX device showing the deployed trocar blade (TB) after advancement of the trocar (T) from the catheter sheath and the inflated 8-mm anchor balloon (AB) and 10 mm dilating balloon (DB). A second guidewire exits from a side guidewire port (GW). (*Courtesy of* Boston Scientific, Inc., Marlborough, MA; with permission.)

accidental loss of cyst access and to maintain apposition of the cyst wall against the bowel wall. After removal of the trocar, the cyst contents are aspirated, contrast may be injected, and the first guidewire is inserted through the catheter, while keeping the anchor balloon inflated. Two standard 0.035-inch guidewires can then be inserted through the separately labeled ports at the handle end of the exchange-free device.

PSEUDOCYST VERSUS WALLED-OFF NECROSIS

What has been ignored thus far in this article is the importance of PFC contents in determining the ultimate methods and success of intervention. Proper distinction between pancreatic pseudocysts and walled-off necrosis (WON) dictates the most appropriate therapeutic approach, because WON may require multiple procedures and more intensive drainage techniques. Inappropriate management of WON as a pseudocyst can result in significant complications.[19] Innovations in the endoscopic management of WON have focused on the use of larger bore metal stents (also applied to pseudocyst drainage) and pursuit of direct debridement or endoscopic necrosectomy.

NECROSECTOMY

The first case series on endoscopic therapy for pancreatic necrosis by continuous irrigation was reported in 1996.[20] Eleven patients received transgastric drainage of WON. Complete resolution was achieved in 9 patients (81.8%) and complications occurred in 5 patients (45.5%).

The first report of direct endoscopic necrosectomy in 3 patients was in 2000.[21] All 3 patients had failed EUS-guided transmural stenting. Transmural puncture was followed by tract dilation using a 16-mm balloon to achieve "fenestration" of the gastric wall. Aggressive debridement of necrosis was performed under direct endoscopy with various off-the-shelf extraction tools including baskets and snares. Weekly debridement was performed until resolution of necroses. There were no serious complications.

SELF-EXPANDABLE METAL STENTS

As an alternative to aggressive balloon catheter dilation of the cystenterostomy tract, direct endoscopic necrosectomy may also be facilitated by placement of a large diameter metal stent. Apart from creating a channel large enough to perform direct endoscopic necrosectomy, multiple additional theoretic advantages have driven the employment of self-expandable metal stents (SEMS) in the management of PFCs. The substantially larger lumen diameter of a SEMS should improve drainage and reduce rates of stent occlusion, thereby decreasing recurrences and secondary infections. A SEMS may also reduce the risk of leakage between the cyst and enteric lumens when these are inadequately adherent. A tamponade effect created by the SEMS may reduce the risk of bleeding from the cystenterostomy. A practical advantage to use of a SEMS is the reduced procedure time resulting from placement of a single stent rather than the placement of multiple plastic stents.

The use of a SEMS to drain a pseudocyst was first introduced in 1994 in a case report of a patient who had failed several attempts at nasocystic drainage of an infected pseudocyst.[22] Because covered SEMS were not available at the time, a 10 mm × 4.5 cm uncovered SEMS was placed and left in place permanently. In 2008, EUS-guided placement of a fully covered SEMS (FCSEMS) was reported in 18 patients with PFCs.[23] The patients had not undergone previous treatment attempts. The authors inserted a 10 mm × 60 mm biliary FCSEMS (Viabil; Conmed, Utica, NY) as well as a 10F plastic stent either alongside (n = 4) or through (n = 14) the SEMS lumen to prevent migration. The technical and clinical (complete resolution of fluid collections) success rates were high at 95% and 75%, respectively. However, there was a high complication rate of more than 40%, including one internal stent migration. The use of a 10-mm biliary FCSEMS (Wallstent, Boston Scientific, Marlborough, MA) was also reported in a patient with an abscess that failed double-pigtail stent and irrigation through a nasocystic catheter.[24] The stent was placed transduodenally and the abscess resolved. The stent was easily removed with a snare 4 weeks later.

Esophageal FCSEMS with larger lumen diameters than biliary FCSEMS were later used to treat PFCs. A 22-mm covered esophageal FCSEMS (Alimaxx-E, Merit Medical Systems, Inc., South Jordan, UT) with a 27-mm flare was used to drain WON that had failed 4 prior necrosectomy sessions with plastic stenting.[25] The larger FCSEMS was placed alongside a previously inserted plastic stent and a Foley irrigation catheter. The FCSEMS was removed 2 weeks after placement and the WON subsequently resolved. In another report, partially covered SEMS with diameters of 20 to 25 mm and a length of 5 cm (Leufen, Achen, Germany) were inserted through the scope for drainage of WON in 3 patients.[26] In all patients, it was possible to enter the cyst through the SEMS with an upper endoscope to perform additional endoscopic necrosectomy. Removal of all necroses was accomplished after 2 to 3 procedures. The cysts resolved in all patients. There were no migrations.

In 2012, our group reported on the use of a conventional 10 × 40-mm biliary FCSEMS (Wallflex; Boston Scientific) for the treatment of pseudocysts with indeterminate adherence.[27] The FCSEMS was placed without prior tract dilation to minimize any risk of leakage or perforation (**Fig. 4**). FCSEMS placement was technically successful in all patients without complications. The FCSEMS was removed 7 to 10 days after insertion and we observed formation of a mature tract with fusion of the cyst and GI tract. The FCSEMS was exchanged for two or three 10F × 3 cm long double-pigtail stents and left in situ for spontaneous extrusion. For PFCs that contained necroses and required debridement, we balloon dilated the tract to 12 to 15 mm followed by endoscopic debridement with an adult gastroscope. In 1 patient,

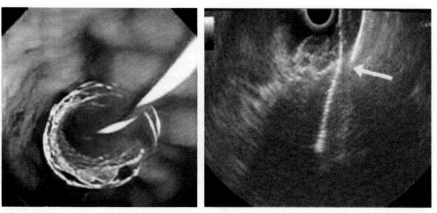

Fig. 4. Biliary fully covered self-expanding metal stent (10 mm × 4-cm) deployed for drainage of a nonadherent pseudocyst. The *arrow* shows the "waist" with bow-tie configuration where the stent traverses the bowel wall.

cystenterostomy dilation resulted in dehiscence and was treated with repeat FCSEMS placement. Cyst resolution was achieved in 78% of patients.

LIMITATION OF LUMINAL STENTS FOR TRANSLUMINAL DRAINAGE

Conventional luminal stents are tubular in form, conceived for coaxial placement within a lumen for relief of an obstruction owing to a malignant or benign stricture. Tubular stents—plastic or metal—have several design deficiencies for transluminal drainage. First, they do not have a mechanism to anchor 2 lumens together. Leakage of contents is possible if physical separation of the lumens occurs. Second, owing to the absence of an anchoring mechanism, stent migration may occur, particularly in the absence of a stricture to hold the stent in place. Premature stent migration can lead to complications, some fatal.[28] Third, the length of tubular stents is greater than that required to span shorter transluminal anastomosis. The exposed stent ends jut into organ or cyst lumens and may cause tissue trauma with resultant perforation or bleeding. Fourth, the excessive length of tubular stents predispose them to clogging from cyst debris or food residue. Finally, if a necrosectomy is required after drainage by plastic stents, the endoscopist must first remove the stents to drive the scope through the transmural tract to extract the necrotic material. This maneuver usually requires aggressive tract dilation. Despite these significant limitations, tubular luminal stents have been used off-label for the drainage of pseudocysts for more than 2 decades.

Alternative stent designs have been pursued to address the weaknesses of conventional stents. In attempt to prevent migration, through-the-scope deployment of an 18 × 60-mm, fully covered esophageal nitinol SEMS with "antimigratory" 26-mm diameter flared flanges (Niti-S; Taewoong-Medical Co, Ilsan, Korea) was used in a series in 10 patients.[29] Despite the antimigratory flanges, stent migration occurred in 10% of cses. In a second smaller series of 5 patients, a double pigtail stent was inserted through the stent lumen to prevent migration.[30] Follow-up data on the migration rate was not provided.

LUMEN-APPOSING METAL STENTS

The lumen-apposing metal stent (LAMS) for transluminal drainage was invented and patented by Binmoeller in 2004 (US patent 8,425,539, filed April 12, 2004) and first reported in animal studies in 2011.[31] It was designed to overcome many of the shortcomings of tubular stents. The inventor named the LAMS "AXIOS" to capture 2 key features of the stent: axial deployment and creation of a transluminal anastomosis (*axial ostomy*).

The AXIOS is a nitinol braided FCSEMS with bilateral double walled flanges in a dumbbell configuration that are perpendicular to the lumen and hold the tissue walls in apposition to create an anastomosis (**Fig. 5**). Fully expanded, the stent's flanges are approximately twice that of its mid-lumen diameter (20 mm diameter flanges for a 10-mm LAMS and 24 mm flanges for a 15-mm LAMS). The bilateral flanges are designed to reduce stent migration and approximate structures to reduce rates of perforation and leak. Furthermore, the flanges are short in length and, therefore, have limited extension into the gastrointestinal tract lumen and fluid collection cavity, potentially reducing the risk of stent erosion.

LUMEN-APPOSING METAL STENT DELIVERY SYSTEM

The short, 1-cm length of the LAMS mandates precise deployment across the cyst and bowel walls. The delivery system of the AXIOS was designed for this requirement.

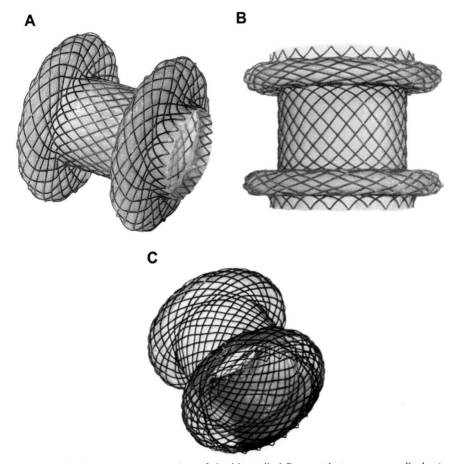

Fig. 5. (*A–C*) The AXIOS stent consists of double-walled flanges that are perpendicular to the lumen and hold the tissue walls in apposition.

The handle of the AXIOS delivery system is Luer locked onto the echoendoscope instrumentation channel inlet port, similar to a standard fine needle aspiration needle (**Fig. 6**). This attachment enables single operator, single-hand control for the entire stent delivery.

The delivery system handle consists of a distal portion (black hub) for catheter control and a proximal portion (gray hub) for stent control (**Fig. 7**). The 10.8F catheter is advanced into the fluid collection by manipulation of the black hub and then locked into position. To deploy the stent, the yellow safety clip is removed from the stent lock. Retraction of the gray hub to a halfway point results in unsheathing of the distal stent flange within the collection cavity for distal flange release. There is a full stop at the halfway point and a "click" is heard as the stent deployment hub locks into place. Complete deployment of the distal flange is verified under sonographic imaging control. The black catheter control hub is then unlocked and retracted until the point at which the distal stent flange starts to compress against the wall of the collection cavity. After relocking the catheter control hub, the stent deployment hub is then completely retracted and the proximal stent flange is unsheathed and the flange deployed within the echoendoscope working channel (**Fig. 8**). The proximal flange, already deployed in the echoendoscope working channel, is then released by advancement of the catheter hub while simultaneously retracting the echoendoscope away from the bowel wall.

Several features were integrated into the catheter sheath to allow multi-imaging control of stent deployment. A 1-cm black band at the distal end of the white catheter sheath indicates the position of the preloaded proximal flange, compressed inside the catheter sheath (**Fig. 9**). The proximal flange can be deployed under direct endoscopic visualization by pulling back the white catheter sheath until visualization of at least 2 to 3 mm of the black band occurs. Once the catheter is pulled back enough, fully retracting the gray stent deployment hub deploys the proximal flange into the bowel lumen. The catheter sheath also has 2 radiopaque markers indicating each end of the preloaded stent to enable fluoroscopic control of stent position. It should be noted, however, that the use of fluoroscopy for routine stent deployment is not needed. Switching from EUS imaging to fluoroscopic guidance is not recommended because this change risks a shift in and loss of the optimal sonographic access plane. It also results in unnecessary radiation exposure.

ELECTROCAUTERY ENHANCED DELIVERY SYSTEM

Initially, delivery of the AXIOS required multiple over-the-wire device exchanges according to the Seldinger technique. Access to the cyst was first obtained with a 19-G

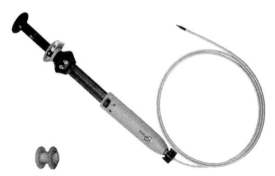

Fig. 6. The AXIOS stent delivery system. (*Courtesy of* Boston Scientific, Inc., Marlborough, MA; with permission.)

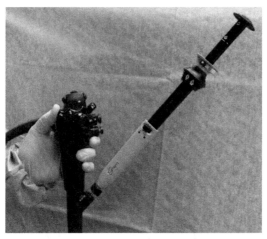

Fig. 7. The handle of the AXIOS delivery system is Luer locked onto the echoendoscope instrumentation channel inlet port, analogous to a standard fine needle aspiration needle. The handle consists of a distal portion for catheter control and a proximal portion for stent control. (*Courtesy of* Boston Scientific, Inc., Marlborough, MA; with permission.)

fine needle aspiration needle, followed by contrast injection to define cyst anatomy for guidewire placement into the cavity. The needle was then exchanged for a dilating balloon to expand ("prime") the cyst puncture tract for delivery catheter insertion. Finally, the dilating catheter was exchanged for the AXIOS catheter delivery system.

As with the technique for any type of metal stent deployment, each step of this process was an opportunity for technical complication. In response, Binmoeller

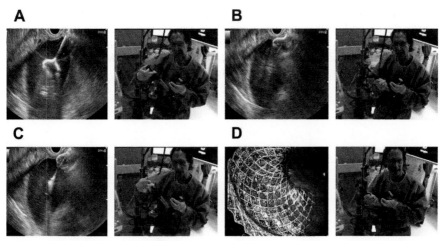

Fig. 8. Deployment of a lumen-apposing metal stents into a peripancreatic fluid collection. (*A*) The stent is advanced into the collection. The gray hub retraction to a halfway point unsheathes the distal flange within the collection. (*B*) The black hub is retracted until the stent compressions the collection cavity wall. (*C*) The gray hub is fully retracted to unsheathe the proximal flange, deploying it within the echoendoscope working channel. (*D*) The black hub is advanced while retracting the echoendoscope away from the bowel wall to release the proximal flange.

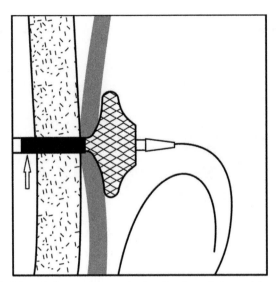

Fig. 9. A 1-cm black band allows endoscopic visualization of the position of the preloaded AXIOS stent within the delivery catheter.

developed the "hot" AXIOS, an electrocautery-enhanced delivery system that enables the operator to access the cyst lumen with a LAMS-loaded catheter followed by immediate deployment of the LAMS. The risk of leakage is reduced if not eliminated because the tract remains sealed off after puncture by the 10.8F delivery catheter until LAMS deployment. Importantly, the need for Seldinger over-the-wire exchange is eliminated. The tamponade effect of the fully covered LAMS reduces the risk of clinically relevant bleeding from the transmural tract.

The hot AXIOS device integrates cautery into the nosecone at the catheter tip. Two radially distributed diathermic wires converge around the guidewire lumen to optimize current density to provide a clean, sharp cut with minimal coagulation effect (**Fig. 10**). Cautery enables transmural advancement of the LAMS delivery catheter into the target lumen without preliminary tract dilation.

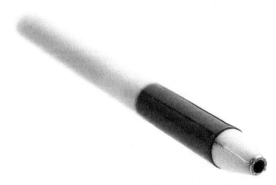

Fig. 10. Tip of the 10.8-F AXIOS catheter. Two radially distributed diathermic wires converge around the guidewire lumen. The catheter houses the AXIOS stent for immediate deployment after entry into the target lumen. (*Courtesy of* Boston Scientific, Inc., Marlborough, MA; with permission.)

SUMMARY

The LAMS is the first stent specifically designed for EUS-guided transluminal drainage of extraintestinal fluid collections. Together with the "hot" electrocautery-enhanced delivery system, this platform marks the most recent evolutionary stage of endoscopic therapy of PFCs. In the last 4 decades, management has progressed from the first attempt at drainage by simple but ineffectual pseudocyst aspiration, to single-device, single maneuver deployment of a LAMS. The LAMS platform has made endoscopic drainage of PFCs easier and safer, while serving as a port for safe entry into the cyst cavity to extend the reach of endoscopic diagnosis and therapy. Tools conceived for EUS-guided transluminal intervention have emerged and are opening the door to new frontiers of endoscopic transluminal therapy.

REFERENCES

1. Rogers BH, Cicurel NJ, Seed RW. Transgastric needle aspiration of pancreatic pseudocyst through an endoscope. Gastrointest Endosc 1975;21(3):133–4.
2. Hancke S, Pedersen JF. Percutaneous puncture of pancreatic cysts guided by ultrasound. Surg Gynecol Obstet 1976;142(4):551–2.
3. Shetty AN. Pseudocysts of the pancreas: an overview. South Med J 1980;73(9): 1239–42.
4. Kozarek RA, Brayko CM, Harlan J, et al. Endoscopic drainage of pancreatic pseudocysts. Gastrointest Endosc 1985;31(5):322–7.
5. Tyberg A, Karia K, Gabr M, et al. Management of pancreatic fluid collections: a comprehensive review of the literature. World J Gastroenterol 2016;22(7): 2256–70.
6. Sahel J, Bastid C, Pellat B, et al. Endoscopic cystoduodenostomy of cysts of chronic calcifying pancreatitis: a report of 20 cases. Pancreas 1987;2(4):447–53.
7. Cremer M, Deviere J, Engelholm L. Endoscopic management of cysts and pseudocysts in chronic pancreatitis: long-term follow-up after 7 years of experience. Gastrointest Endosc 1989;35(1):1–9.
8. Binmoeller KF, Seifert H, Walter A, et al. Transpapillary and transmural drainage of pancreatic pseudocysts. Gastrointest Endosc 1995;42(3):219–24.
9. Smits ME, Rauws EA, Tytgat GN, et al. The efficacy of endoscopic treatment of pancreatic pseudocysts. Gastrointest Endosc 1995;42(3):202–7.
10. Grimm H, Binmoeller KF, Soehendra N. Endosonography-guided drainage of a pancreatic pseudocyst. Gastrointest Endosc 1992;38(2):170–1.
11. Wiersema MJ. Endosonography-guided cystoduodenostomy with a therapeutic ultrasound endoscope. Gastrointest Endosc 1996;44(5):614–7.
12. Wiersema MJ, Baron TH, Chari ST. Endosonography-guided pseudocyst drainage with a new large-channel linear scanning echoendoscope. Gastrointest Endosc 2001;53(7):811–3.
13. Seewald S, Ang TL, Kida M, et al. EUS 2008 Working Group document: evaluation of EUS-guided drainage of pancreatic-fluid collections (with video). Gastrointest Endosc 2009;69(2 Suppl):S13–21.
14. Kruger M, Schneider AS, Manns MP, et al. Endoscopic management of pancreatic pseudocysts or abscesses after an EUS-guided 1-step procedure for initial access. Gastrointest Endosc 2006;63(3):409–16.
15. Lopes CV, Pesenti C, Bories E, et al. Endoscopic-ultrasound-guided endoscopic transmural drainage of pancreatic pseudocysts and abscesses. Scand J Gastroenterol 2007;42(4):524–9.

16. Ahlawat SK, Charabaty-Pishvaian A, Jackson PG, et al. Single-step EUS-guided pancreatic pseudocyst drainage using a large channel linear array echoendoscope and cystotome: results in 11 patients. JOP 2006;7(6):616–24.
17. Reddy DN, Gupta R, Lakhtakia S, et al. Use of a novel transluminal balloon accessotome in transmural drainage of pancreatic pseudocyst (with video). Gastrointest Endosc 2008;68(2):362–5.
18. Binmoeller KF, Smith I, Gaidhane M, et al. A kit for EUS-guided access and drainage of pancreatic pseudocysts: efficacy in a porcine model. Endosc Ultrasound 2012;1(3):137–42.
19. Baron TH, Harewood GC, Morgan DE, et al. Outcome differences after endoscopic drainage of pancreatic necrosis, acute pancreatic pseudocysts, and chronic pancreatic pseudocysts. Gastrointest Endosc 2002;56(1):7–17.
20. Baron TH, Thaggard WG, Morgan DE, et al. Endoscopic therapy for organized pancreatic necrosis. Gastroenterology 1996;111(3):755–64.
21. Seifert H, Wehrmann T, Schmitt T, et al. Retroperitoneal endoscopic debridement for infected peripancreatic necrosis. Lancet 2000;356(9230):653–5.
22. Maisin JM, Bradette M, Buscail L, et al. Patency of endoscopic cystoduodenostomy maintained by a Z stent. Gastrointest Endosc 1994;40(6):765–8.
23. Talreja JP, Shami VM, Ku J, et al. Transenteric drainage of pancreatic-fluid collections with fully covered self-expanding metallic stents (with video). Gastrointest Endosc 2008;68(6):1199–203.
24. Tarantino I, Traina M, Barresi L, et al. Transgastric plus transduodenal necrosectomy with temporary metal stents placement for treatment of large pancreatic necrosis. Pancreas 2010;39(2):269–70.
25. Antillon MR, Bechtold ML, Bartalos CR, et al. Transgastric endoscopic necrosectomy with temporary metallic esophageal stent placement for the treatment of infected pancreatic necrosis (with video). Gastrointest Endosc 2009;69(1):178–80.
26. Belle S, Collet P, Post S, et al. Temporary cystogastrostomy with self-expanding metallic stents for pancreatic necrosis. Endoscopy 2010;42(6):493–5.
27. Weilert F, Binmoeller KF, Shah JN, et al. Endoscopic ultrasound-guided drainage of pancreatic fluid collections with indeterminate adherence using temporary covered metal stents. Endoscopy 2012;44(8):780–3.
28. Martins FP, Rossini LG, Ferrari AP. Migration of a covered metallic stent following endoscopic ultrasound-guided hepaticogastrostomy: fatal complication. Endoscopy 2010;42(Suppl 2):E126–7.
29. Attam R, Trikudanathan G, Arain M, et al. Endoscopic transluminal drainage and necrosectomy by using a novel, through-the-scope, fully covered, large-bore esophageal metal stent: preliminary experience in 10 patients. Gastrointest Endosc 2014;80(2):312–8.
30. Saxena P, Singh VK, Messallam A, et al. Resolution of walled-off pancreatic necrosis by EUS-guided drainage when using a fully covered through-the-scope self-expandable metal stent in a single procedure (with video). Gastrointest Endosc 2014;80(2):319–24.
31. Binmoeller KF, Shah J. A novel lumen-apposing stent for transluminal drainage of nonadherent extraintestinal fluid collections. Endoscopy 2011;43(4):337–42.

Endoscopic Ultrasound–Guided Drainage of Pancreatic Fluid Collections

Marc Giovannini, MD

KEYWORDS

- Pancreatic abscess • Pancreatic pseudocyst • Therapeutic echoendoscope
- EUS-guided drainage

KEY POINTS

- The EUS guided approach is now regarded as the best option for the drainage of pancreatic fluid collections.
- EUS drainage of pancreatic fluid collections has clinical efficacy similar to surgical or percutaneous approaches but with lower morbidity and lower costs.
- The large diameter of lumen-apposing stents has created an acceptable alternative for the drainage of pancreatic necrosis – direct endoscopic necrosectomy.

 Video content accompanies this article at http://www.giendo.theclinics.com.

INTRODUCTION

The management of pancreatic pseudocysts (PPCs) has traditionally been surgical. Although highly effective, surgery may be associated with a complication rate of 35% and a mortality of 10%.[1] This has encouraged the development of nonsurgical approaches. Percutaneous puncture and aspiration under ultrasonography or CT guidance has been used, but aspiration alone has been found ineffective due to high recurrence rates of up to 71%.[2] Continuous percutaneous drainage with indwelling catheters reduces the relapse rates but may be associated with a complication rate ranging from 5% to 60%. Complications include fistula formation, infection, and bleeding.

Endoscopic transmural drainage of PPC is an alternative nonsurgical approach. Since the first reports by Sahel and colleagues[3] and Cremer and colleagues,[4] endoscopic drainage of PPCs has become established. This entails the creation of a fistulous tract between the PPC and the gastric lumen (cystogastrotomy) or duodenal lumen (cystoduodenostomy). Having established endoscopic access to the PPC, a

Medico-Surgical Digestive Oncology, Paoli-Calmettes Institute, 232 Boulevard de Sainte-Marguerite, Marseille 13009, France
E-mail address: uemco@ipc.unicancer.fr

Gastrointest Endoscopy Clin N Am 28 (2018) 157–169
https://doi.org/10.1016/j.giec.2017.11.004
1052-5157/18/© 2017 Elsevier Inc. All rights reserved.

nasocystic catheter or a stent can be placed for continuous drainage. The obvious limitation of endoscopic transmural drainage of PPC was its relatively blind approach. The risk of perforation is particularly high when endoscopically visible intraluminal bulging was absent. A major risk of endoscopic cystoduodenostomy or cystogastrostomy is hemorrhage (6% of cases).[3,4]

Endoscopic ultrasound (EUS)-guided drainage is now firmly established as the best option for drainage of pancreatic fluid collections (PFCs). It has high clinical efficacy, similar to surgical and percutaneous approaches but with lower morbidity and costs. It is superior to non–EUS-guided approaches because even collections without endoluminal bulging can be successfully drained.[5–7]

Infected pancreatic and peripancreatic necrosis in acute pancreatitis is potentially lethal, with mortality rates up to 35%. Therefore, there is growing interest in minimally invasive treatment options, such as (EUS-guided) endoscopic transgastric necrosectomy. Transmural drainage alone is sufficient for pseudocysts, but in the context of walled-off necrosis (WON), adjunctive direct endoscopic necrosectomy (DEN) may be required. Traditionally, double-pigtail plastic stents (PSs) were used for transmural drainage, but recently lumen appositioning metallic stents (LAMSs) customized for PFC drainage have become available and are increasingly used, especially in the management of WON, because the larger-diameter stent facilitates drainage and insertion of an endoscope into the WON cavity for DEN.

Increased understandings of the condition have also led to refinements in the definitions in the updated Atlanta classification. This review aims to provide an overview on the management of peri-PFCs, with focus on newer endoscopic interventions.

BASIC PRINCIPLES

PPCs are reported to complicate between 10% and 20% of patients with acute and chronic pancreatitis.[8] A majority of these PPCs are asymptomatic and do not require treatment. Spontaneous regression of PPC is reported to occur in 7% to 60%. The indication for PPC drainage differs depending on whether a cyst develops in the setting of acute or chronic pancreatitis. For PPCs that complicate acute pancreatitis, drainage is indicated when pancreatitis fails to resolve with conservative measures. PPCs that are not associated with persistent pancreatitis should be observed, because there is a high probability of spontaneous resolution. A 6-week observation period is generally recommended before considering decompression. Spontaneous regression after persistence of more than 6 weeks is considered by some to be unlikely. But actually, this cutoff time of 6 weeks is heavily doubted in the literature now and large pseudocyst (>4 cm of size) should be treated.

For PPCs complicating chronic pancreatitis, drainage is indicted to relieve symptoms associated with a space-occupying mass, including neighboring organ compression. Such patients have chronic cysts that remain unchanged over a period of months. Patients typically complain of a dull and constant pain and may develop symptoms of gastric outlet obstruction or jaundice from bile duct compression.

Multiple or multiloculated PPCs sometimes cannot be adequately treated by an endoscopic approach and warrant surgical resection. An endoscopic approach contaminates the cyst and risks infection if the contents of the PPC cannot be completely drained.

The Atlanta classification published in 1992 had been the most used classification system for acute pancreatitis. In 2012, a revised classification system by the acute pancreatitis working group was published.[8] The most notable difference is the recognition that pancreatic necrosis can exist in both acute and chronic forms, the latter now defined as WON (**Table 1**). According to the 2012 updated classification, different

Table 1
Atlanta classification of pancreatic collection revised in 2012

Type of Collection	Time (wk)	Location	Imaging Appearance
Interstitial edematous pancreatitis			
Acute peri-PFC	≤4	Adjacent to pancreas, extrapancreatic only	Homogeneous, fluid attenuation, no liquefaction, not encapsulated
Pseudocyst	>4	Adjacent or distant to pancreas	Homogeneous, fluid attenuation, no liquefaction, encapsulated
Necrotizing pancreatitis			
Acute necrotic collection	≤4	In parenchyma and/or extrapancreatic	Heterogeneous, nonliquefied material, variably loculated, not encapsulated
WON	>4	In parenchyma and/or extrapancreatic	Heterogeneous, nonliquefied material, variably loculated, encapsulated

Data from Banks PA, Bollen TL, Dervenis C, et al. Classification of acute pancreatitis–2012: revision of the Atlanta classification and definitions by international consensus. Gut 2013;62:102–11.

terms have been defined as acute peri-PFC occurring in interstitial edematous pancreatitis, PPC as a delayed (usually more than 4 weeks) complication of interstitial edematous pancreatitis, acute necrotic collection in the early phase before demarcation in necrotizing pancreatitis, and WON surrounded by a radiologically identifiable capsule, which typically develops after 4 weeks from the onset of pancreatitis.

EUS-guided drainage is not advised in the early phase of collection formation due to the lack of a well-circumscribed cyst wall. The differentiation between PPC and WON is also important because endoscopic drainage of WON had been demonstrated to have significantly lower success rates, higher adverse events, more frequent reinterventions, and longer hospital stays.

MATERIAL USED
Interventional Echoendoscopes

Around 1990, Pentax (Argenteuil, France) developed an electronic convex curved linear array echoendoscope (FG 32UA) with an imaging plane in the long axis of the device that overlaps with the instrumentation plane. This echoendoscope, equipped with a 2.0-mm working channel, enabled fine-needle biopsy under EUS guidance. The small working channel of the FG-32UA, however, was a drawback for pseudocyst drainage because it necessitated the exchange of the echoendoscope for a therapeutic duodenoscope to insert either a stent or nasocystic drain. To enable stent placement using an echoendoscope, the EUS interventional echoendoscopes (EG-38UTK) were developed by Pentax-Hitachi (Argenteuil, France). EG38-UTK has a large working channel of 3.8 mm with an elevator allowing the placement of a 10F stent.

Olympus (Rungis, France) has also developed convex array echoendoscopes. The GF-UC30P has a biopsy channel of 2.8 mm, which enables the placement of a 7F stent or nasocystic catheter, and the instrument is equipped with an elevator. And the GF-UCT140 (Olympus Europa) has a larger working-channel of 3.7 mm, allowing the placement of 10F stent. The main drawback of convex linear array echoendoscopes is the more limited imaging field (140° using the Pentax and 180° using the Olympus) produced by an electronic transducer.

Fuji (Montigny-le-Bretonneux, France) has commercialized recently a new therapeutic linear echoendoscope EG-530UT2 with a 3.8-mm working channel.

Needles and Accessories for Pancreatic Pseudocyst Drainage

Electrocautery or nonelectrocautery dilation catheters are currently used as fistula dilation devices for EUS-guided drainage of PPC; however, few studies have investigated the safety and advantages of electrocautery dilation catheters for EUSTD (endoscopic ultrasound guided transmural dilation).

The nonelectrocautery technique consists of puncturing the cyst cavity using a 19-gauge EUS needle, allowing the passage of a 0.035-in guide wire; then, different dilation catheters could be used as an MTW cannula (MTW Endoskopie, Dusseldorf, Germany) followed by a 6F to 10F Soehendra Biliary Dilation Catheter (Cook Medical, Charenton-le-Pont, France) and/or an 8 mm-diameter balloon bile duct dilation catheter.

The electrocautery technique consists of puncturing the cyst directly using the 10F Cystostome (Cook Medical); the first step is the insertion of the needle-knife under EUS guidance into the cavity, then the metallic part of the needle-knife is removed and a 0.035-in guide wire inserted. The second step is the insertion of the 10F part of the Cystostome on the guide wire to create a large opening and allowing the insertion of a second 0.035-in guide wire. The tract could be enlarged using an 8-mm or 10-mm balloon dilation and the previous insertion of the 2 guide wires facilitates the introduction of the 2 plastic pigtail stents of 7F or 8.5F.

DESCRIPTION OF PROCEDURE
Technique of Endoscopic Ultrasound–Guided Drainage Using Plastic Stents

EUS-guided PPC drainage is performed under general anesthesia in the fluoroscopy suite with the patient in the left lateral or prone position (**Fig. 1**). The patient should receive broad-spectrum antibiotics during and after the procedure to reduce the risk of PPC infection. CT-angiography should be performed immediately before the intervention. It gives information more easily than an endoscopic procedure gives about important anatomic details (eg, varices, arterial pseudoaneurysms, multiple cysts or extended necrosis, ascitis, large or atypically located gall bladder, and pleural effusion).

The individual steps are as follows:

1. Locate the cyst and the contact zone between the gastric or duodenal wall and the cyst wall.

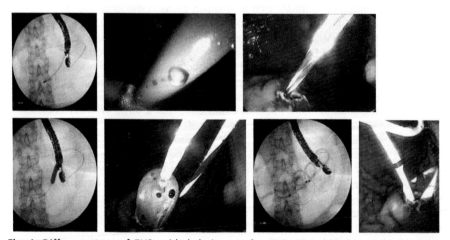

Fig. 1. Different steps of EUS-guided drainage of a PPC using 10F Cystostome + 8-mm balloon dilation followed by the insertion of 2 plastic pigtail stents of 8.5F.

2. The use of Doppler ultrasound to assess the gastric or duodenal wall for interposed vessels is now considered mandatory prior to cyst drainage.
3. Having determined the optimal site for puncture, the PPC is punctured using a 19-gauge fine-needle aspiration needle, and a sample of the cyst contents is aspirated and submitted for biochemical, cytologic, and tumor marker (eg, carcinoembryonic antigen) analysis. If infection is suspected, a sample should be sent for Gram stain and culture and sensitivity or direct puncture of the collection using the needle-knife of the 10F Cystostome.
4. Contrast filling of the PPC under fluoroscopy to document the size and anatomic boundaries of the cyst is not mandatory if a magnetic resonance cholangiopancreatography was previously performed to see a communication of the cyst with the pancreatic duct.
5. The tract is dilated using an 8-mm or 10-mm balloon over the wire or the 8F or 10F Cystostome, allowing the introduction of 2 guide wires.
6. Two stents, 7F or 8.5F (double-pigtail), are placed to drain the PPC or PA.

The choice to insert a nasocystic catheter and a stent for drainage depends on the appearance of the cyst contents. A chronic cyst with clear liquid contents can be drained with an 8.5F or 10F stent alone or with 2 7F stents. An infected cyst mandates irrigation by nasocystic catheter or a 10F stent, and a nasocystic drainage can be placed (see **Fig. 3**). The nasocystic catheter can be removed after 7 days and exchanged for a large-bore stent. Pancreatic cysts complicating necrotizing pancreatitis can be managed endoscopically but require aggressive irrigation and drainage over an extended period time.

Technique of Endoscopic Ultrasound–Guided Drainage Using Lumen Appositioning Metallic Stents

Using NAGI stent or a SPAXUS stent
This stent is constructed from nitinol with a silicone coating specifically designed to act as a temporary cystogastrostomy (see **Fig. 1**; **Figs. 2–4**). The wide flares at both ends of the stent were designed to prevent spontaneous migration. It comes in a variety of lengths (1 cm, 2 cm, and 3 cm) and diameters (10 cm, 12 cm, 14 cm, and 16 mm). A drawstring is present along the gastric flare end of the stent to facilitate removal. To gain access, a 19-gauge needle or a 10F Cystostome is used to puncture the cyst and then a 460-cm 0.035-in guide wire was advanced to form several loops

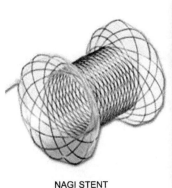

NAGI STENT

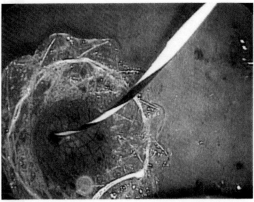

Fig. 2. NAGI stent. (*Courtesy of* TaeWoong Medical, Gyeonggi-do, South Korea; with permission.)

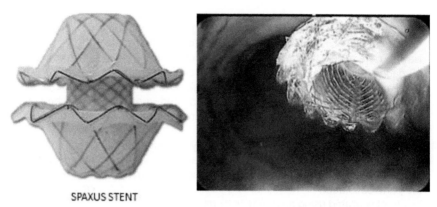

SPAXUS STENT

Fig. 3. SPAXUS stent. (*Courtesy of* TaeWoong Medical, Gyeonggi-do, South Korea; with permission.)

within the cyst under radiological guidance. The tract was predominantly dilated to 8 mm with a graduated balloon device to enable the passage of the stent delivery device through the tract, but no dilatation is required if a 10F Cystostome was used. The introducing device for the stent requires a long wire system and is constrained onto a 10.5F delivery system. A nasocystic catheter was placed through the stent if the PPC was known to be infected or an endoscopic DEN was to be performed.

Using a HOT AXIOS

The deployment of the AXIOS (Boston Scientific, France) stent is characterized by a Luer-Lok (BD, France) mechanism that allows independent deployment of distal and proximal stent anchors. A HOT AXIOS stent comes with an electrocautery wire at the distal tip of the delivery system. The electrocautery tip allows passage of the catheter into the PPC without the need for prior dilation of the tract. It can be advanced along a guide wire that is inserted after initial puncture with a 19-gauge needle, or it can be used to directly access the PFC under EUS guidance.

Multiple Transluminal Gateway Technique

In this technique, the caudal part of the WON was first accessed using EUS guidance, usually from the duodenum or the distal stomach (**Fig. 5**). After dilation of the gut wall

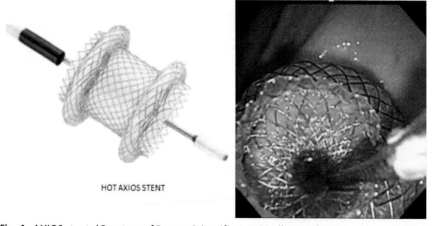

HOT AXIOS STENT

Fig. 4. AXIOS stent. (*Courtesy of* Boston Scientific, Inc, Marlborough, MA; with permission.)

**MULTIPLE
TRANSLUMINAL
GATEWAY TECHNIQUE**

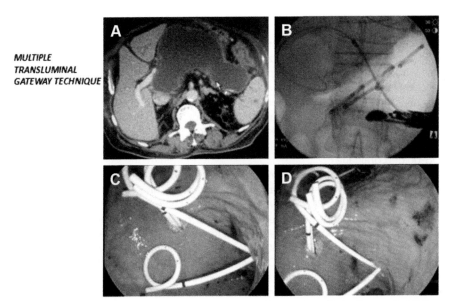

Fig. 5. Multiple gateway technique. (*A*) CT-scan of a patient with walled-off necrosis. (*B*) Fluoroscopic image of EUS-guided access of WON with guide wire coiled within pancreatic collection. (*C, D*) Plastic pigtail stents exiting WON in multiple locations along gastric antrum and body.

and placement of 2 double-pigtail stents of 7F or 8.5 F, multiple sites were created in the WON for placement of additional transmural stents. In general, when the WON was 6 cm to 12 cm in size, only 1 transmural tract was created for transmural drainage; for WON between 12 cm and 15 cm in size, at least 2 transmural tracts were created, and 3 transmural tracts were created for WONs greater than 15 cm. A nasogastric tube was then advanced over a guide wire into the gateway that drained the cranial part of the WON, which was usually at the level of the proximal stomach. As with the standard technique, the nasogastric tube was irrigated to flush out the necrotic debris through the multiple gateways in the stomach.

Technique of Necrosectomy

Two techniques are available (Video 1).

Irrigation technique
After the access session, irrigation necrosectomy sessions were planned at intervals of 2 days to 5 days until most of the nonadherent necrotic material was pushed out and there was clinical improvement of the patient. If necessary to gain a better view, a gastroscope was entered into the cavity, but in a majority of cases this was not necessary. These lavage sessions were performed by flushing SSF (500–1500 mL) through the LAMS using a water-jet system. All the SSF flushed was totally aspirated by suction until the cavity was empty, removing all the nonadherent necrotic debris from the gastric cavity.

Ablative technique
The ablative technique is more aggressive, the goal is to remove the necrosis using snare, Dormia basket, and forceps. This technique is more risky than the irrigation technique and increases the risk of bleeding.

INDICATIONS AND TECHNIQUE

Endosonography is more and more widely used for treatment of PPC.[5–7] This technique allows an operator to locate zones of contact between the cyst and the digestive tract wall. This is especially important when the cyst does not cause extrinsic compression of the organ.

The first point to discuss is when it is necessary to treat a PPC or a pancreatic abscess. PPC and WON must be treated if the collection is symptomatic (pain or fever) or if the lesion remained after 6 weeks of follow-up.

The second point is, what is the best route endoscopic transmural drainage or EUS-guided drainage?

EUS provides real-time ultrasonic guidance of the drainage procedure. Two randomized controlled studies compared EUS-guided with non–EUS-guided endoscopic transmural drainage of PC. EUS was shown to achieve significantly higher success rates. Varadarajulu and colleagues[9] reported a randomized study to compare the rate of technical success between EUS and esophagogastroduodenoscopy (EGD) for transmural drainage of PPCs; 30 patients were randomized to undergo pseudocyst drainage by EUS (n = 15) or EGD (n = 15) over a 6-month period. Except for their gender, there was no difference in patient or clinical characteristics between the 2 cohorts. Although all the patients (n = 14) randomized to an EUS underwent successful drainage (100%), the procedure was technically successful in only 5 of 15 patients (33%) randomized to an EGD (P<.001). All 10 patients who failed drainage by EGD underwent successful drainage of the pseudocyst on a crossover to EUS. There was no significant difference in the rates of treatment success between EUS and EGD after stenting, either by intention-to-treat analysis (100% vs 87%; P = .48) or as-treated analysis (95.8% vs 80%; P = .32). Major procedure-related bleeding was encountered in 2 patients in whom drainage by EGD was attempted; 1 resulted in death and the other necessitated a blood transfusion. No significant difference was observed between EUS and EGD with regard to complications either by intention-to-treat (0% vs 13%; P = .48) or as-treated analyses (4% vs 20%; P = .32). Technical success was significantly greater for EUS than EGD, even after adjusting for luminal compression and gender (adjusted exact odds ratio 39.4; P = .001). Park and colleagues[10] showed the same results (29/31 [94%] vs 21/29 [72%]; P = .0398) with the ability of EUS to visualize PC without endoluminal bulging and guide access to the PC cavity.

One randomized study compared EUS-guided PC drainage with surgical cystogastrostomy.[11] Clinical outcomes between EUS-guided drainage and surgery were similar (success rate: 19/20 [95%] vs 20/20 [100%]; P = .5; complications: 0 vs 2/20 [10%]; P = .24). Patients who underwent EUS-guided drainage, however, had a significantly shorter median hospital stay (2 days vs 6 days; P<.001) and incurred significantly lower mean costs ($7011 vs $15052; P = .003).

Today, EUS should be considered the first-line treatment modality for endoscopic drainage of PPCs given its high technical success rate.

PLASTIC STENT OR LUMEN APPOSITIONING METALLIC STENTS?

LAMSs have larger diameters than PS and may provide more effective drainage. Recent studies that used NAGI (TaeWoong, South Korea), SPAXUS (TaeWoong, South Korea), or AXIOS stents revealed technical success rates that ranged from 91% to 100%.[12–20] Because the treated PFC involved both PC and WON, actual clinical success rates in these series ranged from 77% to 100% (**Table 2**). A randomized study compared LAMSs with PSs for drainage of PC. Both groups achieved technical success in all cases. Median procedure time, however, with

Table 2
Outcomes of patients treated using lumen appositioning metallic stents

Author	Number	Stent Insertion Success (%)	Clinical Success (%)	Pancreatic Pseudocysts	Walled-Off Necrosis	Complication Rate	Type of Stent
Itoi et al,[12] 2013	15	100	100	15	0	1/15	AXIOS
Walter et al,[20] 2015	61	98	90	15	46	8.1%	AXIOS
Shah et al,[19] 2015	33	91	93	22	11	15%	NAGI
Yamamoto et al,[17] 2013	9	100	77	4	5	22%	NAGI
Moon et al,[13] 2014	4	100	100	3	1	0%	SPAXUS
Chandran et al,[18] 2015	48	98.1	76.6	39	9	50%	NAGI
Dhir et al,[15] 2015	47	91.4	87.2	47	0	4.7%	NAGI
Rinninella et al,[14] 2015	93	98.9	93.5	37	56	5.4%	HOT AXIOS

LAMS was significantly shorter than with PS (15.0 vs 29.5 min; $P<.01$). Sharaiha and colleagues.[21] included 230 patients with pseudocysts who received EUS-guided transmural drainage with double-pigtail PSs or fully covered metallic stents. The uses of PSs were associated with lower complete resolution rates (89% vs 98%; $P = .01$) but higher procedural adverse events (31% vs 16%; $P = .006$). On multivariate analysis, the use of PSs was 2.9 times more likely lead to adverse events. Regarding WON, no significant differences in the rates of success, adverse events rates, or procedural costs were observed between the 2 groups.[22] The mean procedure times on initial drainage and reintervention, however, were significantly shorter for the metal stent group.

Four retrospective studies have compared LAMS with PS in the treatment of patients with WON. Mukai and colleagues[22] reported no statistically significant differences in rates of technical success, clinical success, and adverse events between both groups. Mean procedure times for the first EUS-guided drainage and for reintervention, however, were significantly shorter in the LAMS group. There was no statistically significant difference in the total cost between both groups. In contrast, significantly higher success rates with LAMSs were reported by Bapaye and colleagues[23] (94% vs 73.7%; $P<.05$) and Siddiqui and colleagues[24] (95% vs 81%; $P = .001$). Ang and colleagues[25] reported a less frequent need for repeat drainage (34.2% vs 6.3%; $P = .032$) and less frequent need for balloon dilatation prior to DEN and similar costs as PS. Results of these comparative studies are summarized in **Table 3**. But 2 studies are contradictory. Bang and colleagues[26] reported a meta-analysis on 881 patients comparing PS and LAMS for pseudocyst and WON. All published studies from the same period involving PS placement for PFC drainage that included greater than 50 patients; 17 studies met inclusion criteria. No difference was showed for the success, the complication rate, and the recurrence rate **(Table 4)**.

Table 3
Comparative studies of plastic stents versus lumen appositioning metallic stents

	Type of Stent	Clinical Success of Lumen Appositioning Metallic Stents	Clinical Success of Plastic Stents	P
Mukai et al,[22] 2015	LAMS (AXIOS; Niti-S; Hanarostent): 43 PS: 27	97.7%	92.6%	NS
Bapaye et al,[23] 2017	NAGI: 72 PS: 61	94%	73.7%	P<.05
Siddiqui et al,[24] 2017	WallFlex: 121 AXIOS: 86 PS: 106	95% vs 90%	81%	P<.001
Ang et al,[25] 2016	NAGI: 18 PS: 31	Repeat drainage 6.3%	Repeat drainage 34.2%	P<.032

More recently, to compare the clinical outcomes of patients undergoing endoscopic drainage of WON using LAMSs or PSs, a randomized trial (NCT02685865) was initiated by Bang and colleagues.[27] Included in the study were patients with symptomatic WON measuring greater than 6 cm in size and located adjacent to the gastric or duodenal lumen. The total sample size was estimated at 62 patients. An interim audit was performed after 21 patients were randomized (12 LAMSs vs 9 PSs). Stent-related adverse events were observed in 6 of 12 patients randomized to LAMSs compared with none in the PS cohort (50.0 vs 0%; $P = .019$). Three bleedings requiring intensive care unit admissions and blood transfusions; 2 buried stents and 1 biliary compression were also reported. These preliminary observations prompted a change in the study and clinical practice protocols whereby a CT scan was mandatory at 3 weeks in all patients treated with LAMS followed by stent removal if the PFC has resolved.

A randomized study was published by Lee and colleagues[28]; 50 patients (41 men) were included and randomly assigned to either the LAMS group (n = 25) or the PS group (n = 25). The median procedure time with LAMSs was significantly shorter than with PSs (15.0 min vs 29.5 min; $P <.01$). The technical success rate was 100% for both groups. The clinical success rate was 20 of 23 for FCSEMS and 20 of 22 for PSs ($P = .97$). No adverse events occurred in the LAMS group, whereas adverse events occurred in 2 patients in the PS group ($P = .16$). One recurrence was observed during follow-up in the LAMS group and none in the PS group ($P = .15$).

Although LAMS is easier and faster to deploy than PS, it is not indicated for PC drainage, given that it is more costly than PS with a similar clinical success rates. In the context of WON, with the need for more effective drainage, and the potential

Table 4
The success, complication, and the recurrence rates for plastic stents and lumen appositioning metallic stents

	Overall Success Rate (%)	Success Rate for Pancreatic Pseudocysts (%)	Success Rate for Walled-Off Necrosis (%)	Complication Rate (%)	Recurrence Rate (%)
PS	81	85	70	16	10
Metal stent	82	83	78	23	9

Data from Bang JY, Hawes R, Bartolucci A, et al. Efficacy of metal and plastic stents for transmural drainage of pancreatic fluid collections: a systematic review. Dig Endosc 2015;27:486–98.

role for DEN and similar overall costs compared with PS, LAMS should probably be the preferred drainage device but LAMS should be removed quickly as possible to avoid heavy complications, such as bleeding.

ROLE OF ENDOSCOPIC ULTRASOUND–GUIDED NECROSECTOMY IN INFECTED NECROSIS AFTER ACUTE PANCREATITIS

Infected pancreatic and peripancreatic necrosis in acute pancreatitis is potentially lethal, with mortality rates up to 35%. Therefore, there is growing interest in minimally invasive treatment options, such as (EUS-guided) endoscopic transgastric necrosectomy. As with endoscopic transmural drainage of peri-PFCs, the same transluminal access can be expanded to introduce an endoscope through the gastrointestinal wall into the retroperitoneum and remove infected pancreatic necroses under direct visual control. The GEPARD study[29] reported the largest study published; 93 patients (63 men and 30 women; mean age 57 years) underwent a mean of 6 interventions starting at a mean of 43 days after an attack of severe acute pancreatitis. After establishment of transluminal access to the necrotic cavity and subsequent endoscopic necrosectomy, initial clinical success was obtained in 80% of the patients, with a 26% complication and a 7.5% mortality rate at 30 days. After a mean follow-up period of 43 months, 84% of the initially successfully treated patients had sustained clinical improvement, with 10% receiving further endoscopic and 4% receiving surgical treatment of recurrent cavities; 16% suffered recurrent pancreatitis. Same results were recently reported by Brazilian authors[30]; 49 of 56 patients could be successfully treated. DEN was successful in 49 patients (87%) and in 3 (13%) it failed. Mean follow-up was 21 months. During this period, there were 2 (10.5%) pseudocyst recurrences and only 1 (5.2%) recurrence of new episodes of pancreatic necrosis, and all were managed clinically and/or endoscopically. No mortality was related to the procedure. But a retrospective comparison of necrosectomy versus traditional transgastric drainage showed no difference between the 2 techniques[31]; 45 patients were identified who met study criteria: 25 underwent DEN and 20 underwent standard endoscopic drainage. There were no differences in baseline patient or cavity characteristics. Successful resolution was accomplished in 88% who underwent DEN versus 45% who received standard drainage (P<.01), without a change in the total number of procedures. The maximum size of tract dilation was larger in the DEN group (17 mm vs 14 mm; P<.02). Complications were limited to mild periprocedural bleeding with equivalent rates between groups.

Current guidelines suggested that for patients with suspected or confirmed infected necrosis, invasive intervention should be delayed where possible until at least 4 weeks after initial presentation to allow the collection to become walled-off.[32] Percutaneous catheter or endoscopic transmural drainage should be the first step in the treatment of patients with suspected or confirmed (walled-off) infected necrotizing pancreatitis, whereas necrosectomy should be reserved for those who do not improve despite drainage.

SUMMARY

EUS-guided drainage is the first-line modality for drainage of symptomatic PFC. In the context of PC, use of multiple double-pigtail PSs suffices, with high treatment efficacy. This approach provides similar success rates with low complications and better quality of life compared with surgery. LAMS permits more effective drainage with its larger diameter; because of its higher costs than PS, its main role is probably in the context of WON, but the real place and the use of LAMSs should be preceded by more studies to avoid and reduce the risks of complications.

SUPPLEMENTARY DATA

Supplementary data related to this article can be found online at https://doi.org/10.1016/j.giec.2017.11.004.

REFERENCES

1. Kourtesis G, Wilson SE, Williams RA. The clinical significance of fluid collections in acute pancreatitis. Am Surg 1990;56:796–9.
2. Rogers BH, Cicurel NJ, Seed RW. Transgastric needle aspiration of pancreatic pseudocyst through an endoscope. Gastrointest Endosc 1975;21:133–4.
3. Sahel J, Bastid C, Pellat B, et al. Endoscopic cystoduodenostomy of cysts of chronic calcifying pancreatitis : a report of 20 cases. Pancreas 1987;2:447–53.
4. Cremer M, Deviere J, Engelholm L. Endoscopic management of cysts and pseudocysts in chronic pancreatitis : long-term follow-up after 7 years of experience. Gastrointest Endosc 1989;35:1–9.
5. Binmoeller KF, Seifert H, Sohendra N. Endoscopic pseudo-cyst drainage : a new instrument for simplified cystoenterostomy. Gastrointest Endosc 1994;40:112–3.
6. Binmoeller KF, Sohendra N. Diagnosis and treatment of pancreatic pseudocysts. Clin North America 1995;5:805–16.
7. Gerolami R, Giovannini M, Laugier R. Endoscopic drainage of pancreatic pseudocysts guided by endosonography. Endoscopy 1997;29:106–8.
8. Banks PA, Bollen TL, Dervenis C, et al. Classification of acute pancreatitis–2012: revision of the Atlanta classification and definitions by international consensus. Gut 2013;62:102–11.
9. Varadarajulu S, Christein JD, Tamhane A, et al. Prospective randomized trial comparing EUS and EGD for transmural drainage of pancreatic pseudocysts (with videos). Gastrointest Endosc 2008;68(6):1102–11.
10. Park DH, Lee SS, Moon SH, et al. Endoscopic ultrasoundguided versus conventional transmural drainage for pancreatic pseudocysts: a prospective randomized trial. Endoscopy 2009;41:842–8.
11. Varadarajulu S, Lopes TL, Wilcox CM, et al. EUS versus surgical cystgastrostomy for management of pancreatic pseudocysts. Gastrointest Endosc 2008;68:649–55.
12. Itoi T, Nageshwar Reddy D, Yasuda I. New fully-covered self-expandable metal stent for endoscopic ultrasonographyguided intervention in infectious walled-off pancreatic necrosis (with video). J Hepatobiliary Pancreat Sci 2013;20:403–6.
13. Moon JH, Choi HJ, Kim DC, et al. A newly designed fully covered metal stent for lumen apposition in EUS-guided drainage and access: a feasibility study (with videos). Gastrointest Endosc 2014;79:990–5.
14. Rinninella E, Kunda R, Dollhopf M, et al. EUS-guided drainage of pancreatic fluid collections using a novel lumenapposing metal stent on an electrocautery-enhanced delivery system: a large retrospective study (with video). Gastrointest Endosc 2015;82:1039–46.
15. Dhir V, Teoh AY, Bapat M, et al. EUS-guided pseudocyst drainage: prospective evaluation of early removal of fully covered self-expandable metal stents with pancreatic ductal stenting in selected patients. Gastrointest Endosc 2015;82:650–7.
16. Gornals JB, De la Serna-Higuera C, Sanchez-Yague A, et al. Endosonography-guided drainage of pancreatic fluid collections with a novel lumen-apposing stent. Surg Endosc 2013;27:1428–34.

17. Yamamoto N, Isayama H, Kawakami H, et al. Preliminary report on a new, fully covered, metal stent designed for the treatment of pancreatic fluid collections. Gastrointest Endosc 2013;77:809–14.
18. Chandran S, Efthymiou M, Kaffes A, et al. Management of pancreatic collections with a novel endoscopically placed fully covered self-expandable metal stent: a national experience (with videos). Gastrointest Endosc 2015;81:127–35.
19. Shah RJ, Shah JN, Waxman I, et al. Safety and efficacy of endoscopic ultrasound-guided drainage of pancreatic fiuid collections with lumen-apposing covered self-expanding metal stents. Clin Gastroenterol Hepatol 2015;13:747–52.
20. Walter D, Will U, Sanchez-Yague A, et al. A novel lumenapposing metal stent for endoscopic ultrasound-guided drainage of pancreatic fluid collections: a prospective cohort study. Endoscopy 2015;47:63–7.
21. Sharaiha RZ, DeFilippis EM, Kedia P, et al. Metal versus plastic for pancreatic pseudocyst drainage: clinical outcomes and success. Gastrointest Endosc 2015;82:822–7.
22. Mukai S, Itoi T, Baron TH, et al. Endoscopic ultrasound-guided placement of plastic vs. biflanged metal stents for therapy of walled-off necrosis: a retrospective single-center series. Endoscopy 2015;47:47–55.
23. Bapaye A, Dubale NA, Sheth KA, et al. Endoscopic ultrasonography-guided transmural drainage of walled-off pancreatic necrosis: comparison between a specially designed fully covered bi-flanged metal stent and multiple plastic stents. Dig Endosc 2017;29:104–10.
24. Siddiqui AA, Kowalski TE, Loren DE, et al. Fully covered selfexpanding metal stents versus lumen-apposing fully covered self-expanding metal stent versus plastic stents for endoscopic drainage of pancreatic walled-off necrosis: clinical outcomes and success. Gastrointest Endosc 2017;85(4):758–65.
25. Ang TL, Kongkam P, Kwek ABE, et al. A two-center comparative study of plastic and lumen apposing large diameter self-expandable metallic stents in endoscopic ultrasound guided drainage of pancreatic fluid collections. Endosc Ultrasound 2016;5:320–7.
26. Bang JY, Hawes R, Bartolucci A, et al. Efficacy of metal and plastic stents for transmural drainage of pancreatic fluid collections: a systematic review. Dig Endosc 2015;27:486–98.
27. Bang JY, Hasan M, Navaneethan U, et al. Lumen-apposing metal stents (LAMS) for pancreatic fluid collection (PFC) drainage: may not be business as usual. Gut 2017;66(12):2054–6.
28. Lee BU, Song TJ, Lee SS, et al. Newly designed, fully covered metal stents for endoscopic ultrasound (EUS)-guided transmural drainage of peripancreatic fluid collections: a prospective randomized study. Endoscopy 2014;46(12):1078–83.
29. Seifert H, Biermer M, Schmitt W, et al. Transluminal endoscopic necrosectomy after acute pancreatitis: a multicenter study with long-term follow-up (the GEPARD Study). Gut 2009;58(9):1260–6.
30. Coelho D, Ardengh JC, Eulálio JM, et al. Management of infected and sterile pancreatic necrosis by programmed endoscopic necrosectomy. Dig Dis 2008;26(4):364–9.
31. Gardner TB, Chahal P, Papachristou GI, et al. A comparison of direct endoscopic necrosectomy with transmural endoscopic drainage for the treatment of walled-off pancreatic necrosis. Gastrointest Endosc 2009;69(6):1085–94.
32. Working Group IAP/APA Acute Pancreatitis Guidelines. IAP/APA evidence-based guidelines for the management of acute pancreatitis. Pancreatology 2013;13(4 Suppl 2):e1–15.

17. Yamamoto N, Isayama H, Kawakami H, et al. Preliminary report on a new fully covered metal stent designed for the treatment of pancreatic fluid collections. Gastrointest Endosc 2013;77:809–14.

18. Chandran S, Efthymiou M, Kaffes A, et al. Management of pancreatic collections with a novel endoscopically placed fully covered self-expandable metal stent: a national experience (with videos). Gastrointest Endosc 2015;81:127–35.

19. Shah RJ, Shah JN, Waxman I, et al. Safety and efficacy of endoscopic ultrasound-guided drainage of pancreatic fluid collections with lumen-apposing covered self-expanding metal stents. Clin Gastroenterol Hepatol 2015;13:747–52.

20. Walter D, Will U, Sanchez-Yague A, et al. A novel lumen-apposing metal stent for endoscopic ultrasound-guided drainage of pancreatic fluid collections: a prospective cohort study. Endoscopy 2015;47:63–7.

Endoscopic Ultrasound–Guided Biliary Drainage

Brian R. Boulay, MD, MPH[a],*, Simon K. Lo, MD[b]

KEYWORDS

- Endoscopic ultrasound • Biliary drainage • Bile duct stricture
- Rendezvous procedure • Hepaticogastrostomy • Choledochoduodenostomy

KEY POINTS

- EUS-guided biliary drainage provides an alternative to percutaneous or surgical drainage when biliary decompression is needed but conventional ERCP methods fail.
- EUS-BD is performed via an intrahepatic approach or extrahepatic approach. Intrahepatic approach can include either direct hepaticogastrostomy or antegrade biliary access for stent placement, whereas the extrahepatic approach involves either direct choledocho-duodenostomy or endoscopic transduodenal rendezvous procedure.
- EUS-guided biliary drainage succeeds in greater than 90% of cases when performed by experts, but the adverse event rate of greater than 20% remains high.
- The technical complexity and rare opportunity to perform these cases should prompt caution and practice should be limited at this time to expert centers.

INTRODUCTION

The advances of fine-needle technologies, catheter cautery devices, dilators, and metal stents have gradually transformed endoscopic ultrasound (EUS) from merely a diagnostic modality to one that offers therapy over the past two decades. The ability to visualize extraluminal structures, such as the biliary tree, offers therapeutic options previously unavailable for biliary drainage (BD). Although endoscopic retrograde cholangiopancreatography (ERCP) remains the primary method for achieving BD, it is not universally successful. ERCP may fail for numerous reasons, such as failure to reach the papilla for attempted cannulation, or because of technical issues preventing successful navigation of a biliary stricture. Malignant obstruction of the gastric outlet or duodenum may prevent the endoscopist from reaching the papilla, or the biliary orifice may be obscured by a previously placed duodenal stent. A large pancreatic, duodenal, or ampullary tumor may make it impossible to recognize the

[a] Division of Gastroenterology and Hepatology, University of Illinois Hospital and Health Sciences System, 840 S Wood Street, M/C 716, Chicago, IL 60612, USA; [b] Pancreatic and Biliary Disease Program, Digestive Diseases, Cedars Sinai Medical Center, 8700 Beverly Boulevard, South Tower, Suite 7511, Los Angeles, CA 90048, USA
* Corresponding author.
E-mail address: bboulay@UIC.EDU

Gastrointest Endoscopy Clin N Am 28 (2018) 171–185
https://doi.org/10.1016/j.giec.2017.11.005
1052-5157/18/© 2017 Elsevier Inc. All rights reserved.

giendo.theclinics.com

ampullary structures to cannulate the bile duct. The papilla may be hidden within a duodenal diverticulum. The patient may have postsurgical anatomy, such as Billroth II or Roux-en-Y reconstruction, making the papilla difficult to reach and requiring specialized equipment, such as deep enteroscopes and modified cannulotomes. At other times, all the conditions may seem to be in favor of the endoscopist and yet cannulation fails despite all efforts, including specialized techniques, such as pancreatic duct stent placement, double-wire technique, or needle knife papillotomy.

In cases of failed conventional ERCP, patients and endoscopists may elect for a repeat procedure on a later day, referral to a higher level skilled expert for another attempt, or percutaneous BD. EUS-guided BD (EUS-BD) is an emerging technique that combines the advantages of the endoscopic and percutaneous approaches, without the inconveniences and discomfort of an indwelling external catheter. The former options have been the standard treatment of failed ERCP for decades, but since the initial report by Giovannini and coworkers[1] in 2001 there has been growing interest and experience in EUS-BD. Several different EUS-guided techniques have been developed to access the obstructed biliary tree from either the stomach or duodenum, according to the location of the stricture, the anatomy of the patient, and the experience of the endoscopist.

TECHNIQUE

EUS-BD is performed in four different ways. The choice of technique depends on the indication for biliary decompression and nature of the anatomic deterrent from performing the conventional ERCP. An intrahepatic approach is used by accessing the bile duct from the stomach to reach the left-sided intrahepatic ducts. Decompression of the biliary tree can then be performed by either inserting a transgastric hepaticogastrostomy (EUS-HGS) stent or advancing a guidewire across the stricture and the papilla to complete an antegrade stent placement (EUS-AS). An intrahepatic approach is typically used in cases where endoscopic access to the papilla is impeded by gastric outlet obstruction or an obstructing proximal duodenal tumor, or in patients with a surgically altered anatomy. The extrahepatic approach is performed from within the duodenum as either creation of a new fistula or choledochoduodenostomy (EUS-CDS) or EUS-guided rendezvous procedure (EUS-RV). The method of sedation for the patient is left to the discretion of the treating team, although given the technical complexity of the procedure and risk of complications, general anesthesia is largely considered the most appropriate modality. Likewise, the use of preprocedural antibiotics has not been rigorously studied in this patient population, although antibiotics can be used depending on the underlying disorder of the biliary tree (eg, status post liver transplant) and the possibility of incomplete ductal clearance.

Intrahepatic Approach: Endoscopic Ultrasound–Guided Hepaticogastrostomy

EUS-HGS is an appropriate choice for EUS-BD when endoscopic access to the papilla is difficult because of malignant obstruction of the gastric outlet or proximal duodenum, or in cases of postsurgical anatomy, such as an unusual case of difficult-to-negotiate Roux-en-Y or Billroth II reconstructions. Significant ductal dilation within the left lobe of the liver is highly desirable for this procedure because it allows easy recognition and puncture of the biliary tree. Segment three of the liver is well visualized from the gastroesophageal (GE) junction and the dilated ducts within this region are a suitable target for EUS-guided access. EUS-HGS is not appropriate in cases of cancer infiltration of the gastric wall within the planned path of approach to the bile ducts. Massive ascites and coagulopathy are likewise considered contraindications (**Table 1**). EUS-HGS

Table 1	
Indications for EUS-guided biliary drainage	
Papilla Accessible	**Papilla Inaccessible**
Diverticular relationship	Gastric outlet obstruction
Difficult biliary stricture	Postsurgical anatomy
Failure despite prolonged attempts	Ampullary mass obscuring papilla
	Indwelling duodenal stent

should not be attempted when most intrahepatic obstruction involves the right side of the liver, particularly when the stricture occurs at the hepatic bifurcation or higher, because the typical point of access is via the left-sided intrahepatic ducts.

The technique and equipment of EUS-HGS are not standardized, although most experts agree on use of a 19-gauge needle for access across the wall of the proximal gastric body into the left-sided intrahepatic ducts (**Fig. 1**). The optimal site of puncture has been described as a bile duct of greater than 5 mm within a hepatic segment length of 1 to 3 cm.[2] Once the EUS needle has been advanced into the duct, bile is aspirated through the needle to confirm placement. Further removal of bile fluid to relief engorgement of the biliary compartment to reduce intraprocedural and post-procedural bile leak may be performed, although there is no evidence that this maneuver is beneficial. Contrast should be injected into the biliary tree to obtain a cholangiogram to identify and characterize the obstructive process. A guidewire is then advanced into the duct to maintain access and advance across the lesion, if needed. Wire choice depends on the endoscopist, but an 0.035-inch hydrophilic wire is generally favored to minimize shearing of the wire coating against the needle tip during wire manipulation. The large caliber of the wire lends strength and stability to facilitate additional manipulations. The combination of a 22-gauge needle and

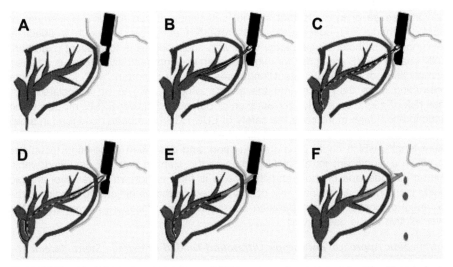

Fig. 1. EUS-guided hepaticogastrostomy. (*A*) The scope is used to identify dilated ducts in the left lobe of the liver. (*B*) The duct is punctured under EUS guidance. (*C*) A wire is advanced into the biliary tree. (*D*) The tract is dilated. (*E*) The stent is inserted across the newly dilated tract. (*F*) Drainage occurs into the stomach through the stent.

0.018-inch guidewire may be used when targeting the bile duct with a stiff 19-gauge needle is not possible, although the smaller needle tract makes subsequent device passage difficult. Additionally, forceful advancement of a catheter device through a tight needle tract risks separation of the liver from the gastric wall, predisposing to significant post-stenting leakage and stent dislodgement. Once the wire is secure within the biliary tree (either coiled within dilated intrahepatic ducts or passed through the obstruction into the duodenum) the needle is withdrawn while the wire maintains access to the biliary tree.

Dilation of the needle tract is then performed to allow creation of the HGS and subsequent stent placement. Dilation may be performed by balloon catheter, graded diameter stiff catheter, or needle knife at the discretion of the endoscopist. This is the critical step that ultimately impacts on the technical success or failure of the drainage procedure. Advancing a common form of biliary catheter or dilator may meet with tremendous tissue resistance even if the initial tract was done with the 19-gauge needle. A firm liver with a tight tract may be pushed away during this process and create a separation of the stomach from the liver, leading to post-procedure bile leak. Outside of the United States, small-caliber wire-guided catheter dilators with a cautery tip are commercially available, and may be used to overcome difficulty in passing instruments through the gastric wall or liver tissue. Conversely, caution must be taken to avoid dilating the tract excessively, because this may increase the risk of bile leak if a plastic stent is used. The use of a needle knife catheter has been linked to the complication of bile leak, and possibly because of the imperfect alignment of the knife tract to that of the wire over which the needle knife is advanced.[3] It may be used cautiously and superficially to widen a gastric opening; however, deep cutting beyond the wall of the stomach should be avoided to prevent perforation, bleeding, or liver laceration. Following dilation, a stent may be advanced over the wire to complete the HGS and allow ongoing BD.

Plastic stents have been used for EUS-HGS but have been largely replaced by partially coated or fully coated self-expanding metallic stents (SEMS) to allow for complete sealing of the HGS tract. However, plastic stents may still be used in benign disease or in ducts that are not sufficiently dilated to allow placement of SEMS. Umeda and colleagues[4] have reported early success with a specially designed 8F catheter single pigtail stent with anchoring flaps to prevent migration. Fully coated SEMS are at risk for migration with ensuing peritonitis, which is a feared complication of EUS-HGS. Stent length seems to be important, with longer stents protruding more than 3 cm into the gastric lumen shown to be associated with less risk of migration and longer duration of patency.[5,6] Newer SEMS models using antimigration flaps to improve the safety of EUS-HGS have been described in small case series.[7] Paik and colleagues[8] have cautioned against choosing an insufficient stent length, which could promote migration, and described a modified technique in which a significant intraluminal portion of the stent is actually deployed within the echoendoscope channel and the scope is then withdrawn under fluoroscopic guidance. Finally, an intrinsic risk of this procedure that is difficult to predict is the potential of post-stenting separation caused by post-procedure movement of the liver relative to the gastric wall.

Intrahepatic Approach: Endoscopic Ultrasound–Guided Antegrade Stent Placement

EUS-AS uses the same technique of accessing the biliary tree via an intrahepatic approach, but instead of stent placement across the newly dilated tract (as in EUS-HGS), the stent is placed across the obstruction itself within the biliary tree. The steps are similar to that of EUS-HGS, although the wire must be passed successfully through the point of obstruction to allow stent placement. This may be difficult in cases of high-grade or eccentrically located strictures where the wire may tend to coil proximal to the stricture. The wire may be manipulated or exchanged to allow passage through the stricture. As in all cases of transmural EUS needle delivery of guidewire, care must be taken to avoid shearing of the wire coating against the sharp needle tip. A small-caliber ERCP catheter should be exchanged for the needle to prevent this from occurring when manipulating the guidewire through the site of obstruction.[9] Following dilation of the tract, the stent delivery system is advanced into the intrahepatic biliary tree and across the obstruction. To minimize transgastric tract dilation and provide long-term biliary decompression, SEMS is the ideal stent to use for this approach. Proper fluoroscopic interpretation of the biliary lesion and identification of the papilla is important to ensure safety and efficacy of stent placement. Some authors suggest use of SEMS long enough to cross both the stricture and ampulla or anastomosis to minimize the chance of postprocedural bile leak through the dilate needle tract. This may occasionally require placement of two overlapping stents to provide sufficient length to bridge the two structures. Following successful therapeutic stenting, a temporary plastic hepaticogastric stent is used to prevent backflow leakage and maintain access for reintervention. To ensure ease of future access, this plastic stent should be straight instead of being a pigtail. Although stent migration across a newly formed tract is not a common issue with EUS-AS, reintervention may be difficult in the setting of incomplete drainage or stent occlusion if the transgastric access tract has been sealed. Alternatively, EUS-AS is combined with EUS-HGS to allow drainage in both directions.[10] The use of SEMS for transpapillary drainage and transgastric drainage may be expensive, without ensuring added clinical benefits.

Extrahepatic Approach: Endoscopic Ultrasound–Guided Choledochoduodenostomy

The choice of EUS-CDS is ideal when there is limited access to the papilla (as with an ampullary tumor) but the extrahepatic bile duct is significantly dilated because of a distal common bile duct obstruction. The duct should be dilated enough to allow puncture with a 19-gauge EUS needle and subsequent stent placement. In this procedure, the linear array echoendoscope is advanced to the duodenal bulb and the dilated common bile duct is punctured at its closest point of approximation to the duodenal wall. Bile is aspirated through the EUS needle to confirm position and a cholangiogram is obtained. The 0.035-inch guidewire is then directed proximally into the intrahepatic biliary tree rather than crossing the distal site of obstruction. The EUS needle is removed while maintaining access with the wire, and the tract is dilated using a balloon catheter or graded dilating catheter. Finally, a plastic stent or fully coated SEMS is placed across the newly created CDS tract. As with EUS-HDS, migration of the SEMS is a known risk factor for postprocedural complications.[11] Lumen-apposing stents have occasionally been used in EUS-CDS procedures, with the largest series to date including 57 patients. The large diameter of the stent requires a significant degree of biliary dilatation for deploying the stent, and most published cases used the smallest size of stent with a 6-mm lumen diameter.[12,13] However, the cautery-assisted delivery system included with the latest generation of lumen-apposing stents can simplify and speed deployment of the stent and achieve BD in appropriate patients.

EUS-CDS is used in cases of duodenal obstruction, as long as the duodenal bulb itself (the site of the planned CDS) is not involved with malignant tissue. If the second or third portion of the duodenum is obstructed, then EUS-CDS is combined with placement of a duodenal stent to relieve the luminal obstruction.

Extrahepatic or Intrahepatic Approach: Endoscopic Ultrasound–Guided Rendezvous

In cases of failed ERCP where the second portion of the duodenum is easily reached but conventional ERCP still fails, EUS-RV is considered as a second-line approach. EUS-RV is always preferred over transmural stenting by either EUS-CDS or EUS-HGS whenever technically feasible, because there is less risk for stent migration, tract dehiscence bile leak, or cholangitis. Additionally, the choice of stents and opportunity for future manipulation favor the use of this modality. Failed transpapillary access caused by a juxtapapillary diverticulum or ampullary cancer may prompt the endoscopist to switch from ERCP to EUS-RV. In this procedure, the dilated intrahepatic or extrahepatic duct is visualized and punctured with the 19-gauge EUS needle, and a long (450 cm) 0.035-inch or 0.025-inch guidewire is then directed downstream through the stenosis and into the duodenum. If the extrahepatic duct is chosen as the site of puncture from a position within the duodenal bulb, then care must be taken to puncture the duct with the needle tip pointing distally toward the papilla rather than proximally into the intrahepatic duct in the retrograde manner (**Fig. 2**). Guidewire manipulation through the papilla is difficult, and procedural time in EUS-RV may be prolonged because of the need to exchange endoscopes.[9] A therapeutic algorithm was recently published where the second portion of the duodenum was shown to be the most effective scope position and first-line strategy for passing the wire downstream and through the papilla in EUS-RV. Guidewire placement from within the second portion of the duodenum requires a short scope position that may be unstable, so if necessary the needle puncture may be performed from the duodenal bulb (with the scope in a coiled or long position) or the proximal stomach (intrahepatic approach with the scope in short position).[14] Once a long length of the wire has been coiled within the

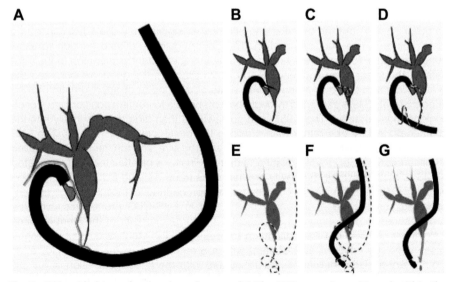

Fig. 2. EUS-guided transduodenal rendezvous. (*A*) The EUS scope is positioned within the duodenal bulb. (*B*) The duct is punctured. (*C*) The wire is advanced into the common duct. (*D*) The wire is manipulated distally across the papilla into the second portion of the duodenum. (*E*) The echoendoscope is removed over the wire. (*F*) A duodenoscope is advanced to the papilla to grasp the wire. (*G*) ERCP proceeds with stent placement for drainage.

duodenum, the echoendoscope is withdrawn leaving the wire in place. A duodeno-scope can then be advanced and the bile duct accessed by cannulating alongside the wire, or by grasping the wire with a grasping forceps or a snare and drawing it into the scope channel. ERCP can then proceed in typical fashion using the access gained by the EUS-RV technique.

CHOICE OF APPROACH

The choice of approach for EUS-BD is left to the endoscopist's discretion based on the indication for EUS-BD. There is no formal consensus for how to decide between intrahepatic or extrahepatic approach, although clinical features of the patient dictate whether some approaches are available (eg, intrahepatic approach may be difficult or impossible when ducts within the left lobe of the liver are nondilated). Therefore the endoscopist must have mastery of multiple techniques to fully use EUS-BD. There is the general impression that an EUS-BD technique that results in transpapillary or antegrade drainage is preferred over transmural creation of a fistula because of a smaller risk of post-procedure bile leak.[15] A prospective randomized trial of EUS-CDS versus EUS-HGS in 49 patients showed no differences in technical or clinical success rates or adverse events between the two techniques, and advised choosing an approach based on endoscopist expertise.[16]

Some have proposed an algorithm for guidance when considering EUS-BD based on patient anatomy or ease of guidewire manipulation. Recently Tyberg and colleagues[17] proposed an algorithm for drainage in which the intrahepatic route was chosen as the initial approach when dilated intrahepatic ducts were seen on cross-sectional imaging and EUS. In this prospective study of 52 patients, EUS-AS was first attempted, with conversion to EUS-HGS if EUS-AS was unsuccessful. Patients with a nondilated intrahepatic duct underwent an extrahepatic approach with EUS-RV as the initial strategy and conversion to EUS-CDS if unsuccessful. When the algorithm was used 52 of 54 patients (96%) underwent technically successful drainage, with more than half of the patients treated by EUS-AS. Adverse events were seen in 10% of patients including one fatal hemorrhage. In 2013 Park and colleagues[18] also proposed an algorithm for EUS-BD based on guidewire manipulation in which 41 of 45 patients (91%) were successfully treated using either EUS-AS or EUS-RV as the initial approach. The limited experience in small case series to date does not allow a formal recommendation. Further evaluations are needed to address this issue.

STENT CHOICE

Data on the choice of plastic versus metallic stents in EUS/BD are limited. When EUS-AS or EUS-RV is used, the stent choice may parallel that of ERCP when considering the cause of the obstruction and the patient's prognosis. When a new permanent fistula is created with EUS-CDS or EUS-HGS, the stent choice is left to the discretion of the endoscopist. Stent patency in SEMS seems to be longer based on a retrospective analysis of patients with EUS-HGS, although plastic stents are available in longer lengths, which may allow for deeper insertion into the biliary system and limit the risk of migration.[19,20] If a plastic stent is chosen, it should generally be the straight stent. A pigtail stent may be able to hold the tract together and is less susceptible to migration, has less effective drainage, and is difficult to exchange to a new one. Tyberg and colleagues[17] described the following factors in choice of stent type: the degree of ductal dilatation, the underlying disease, whether the wire could cross the anastomosis, the length of fistula tract, and surgical candidacy of the patient. Forty-one of the 52 patients in the Tyberg study (79%) received SEMS, whereas 11 patients

(21%) received plastic stents. The preference for SEMS is in accordance with recent studies where the wider lumen and longer patency duration of SEMS make them an attractive choice over plastic stents when reintervention for stent exchange is not desirable.

OUTCOMES

Two recent systematic reviews and meta-analyses have collected the published experience with EUS-BD showing its effectiveness. Wang and colleagues[21] included 42 studies with a total of 1192 patients. The cumulative technical success rate was 94.71%, whereas the functional success rate was 91.66% and the adverse event rate was 23.32%. There were no statistical differences in technical or functional success between the 14 prospective studies and the 28 retrospective studies. There was a statistically higher technical success rate in studies published after 2013, likely reflecting improved technique and experience.

A meta-analysis of 10 of the included studies found no differences in technical or clinical success rates between the intrahepatic or extrahepatic approaches.[21] In contrast, Ikeuchi and Itoi[20] showed superior technical success rates for EUS-HGS (95%) and EUS-CDS (92%) compared with lower rates for EUS-RV (81%) and EUS-AS (77%), although these results did not reach statistical significance. It is interesting that the Ikeuchi and Itoi[20] study had better success rates using the two EUS-BD techniques, which require creation of a new fistula. However, the rate of technical success for EUS-RV and EUS-AS in this review was lower than the corresponding 89.7% and 91.3% noted by Wang and colleagues.[21] A comparison of results for intragastric versus extragastric approaches is shown in **Table 2**.[16,22–25]

The other systematic review conducted by Khan and colleagues[26] included a total of 1186 patients and used a weighted pooled rate (WPR) measurement for technical success (90%) and adverse events (17%). When high-quality studies were analyzed, technical success WPR was 94% and adverse events WPR was 16%, overall consistent with the results from the Wang and colleagues[21] systematic review.

The outcomes of EUS-BD are comparable with that of percutaneous drainage according to recent data. When compared with percutaneous transhepatic biliary drainage (PTBD) in a meta-analysis of nine studies involving 483 patients, EUS-BD was associated with better clinical success (odds ratio [OR], 0.45), fewer adverse events (OR, 0.23), and fewer reinterventions (OR, 0.13). There was no difference in technical success between the two procedures.[27] The authors noted that the EUS-BD procedures were all performed by endoscopic experts, whereas PTBD is much more widely available and routine in current practice.

Table 2					
Comparisons of extrahepatic versus intrahepatic routes for EUS-guided biliary drainage					
Author	Study Design	Success IH	Success EH	AE IH	AE EH
Dhir et al,[22] 2013	Retrospective	16/17 (94%)	18/18 (100%)	4/17 (23.5%)	0
Dhir et al,[23] 2014	Retrospective	34/36 (94%)	31/32 (97%)	11/36 (30%)	3/32 (9%)
Kawakubo et al,[24] 2014	Retrospective	19/20 (95%)	42/44 (95%)	6/20 (30%)	6/44 (14%)
Poincloux et al,[25] 2015	Retrospective	66/71 (94%)	27/30 (93%)	10/71 (14%)	2/30 (7%)
Artifon et al,[16] 2015	Prospective	22/25 (91%)	17/24 (77%)	5/25 (20%)	3/24 (13%)

Abbreviations: AE, adverse events; EH, extrahepatic; IH, intrahepatic.

Adapted from Liao WC, Angsuwatcharakon P, Isayama H, et al. International consensus recommendations for difficult biliary access. Gastrointest Endosc 2017;85(2):295–304; with permission.

SAFETY AND ADVERSE EVENTS

In a recent analysis of the adverse events associated with EUS-BD, the overall rate of events was 23.32%. In this analysis, studies published after 2013 did not have a statistically better rate of adverse events when compared with earlier studies. Common adverse events included bleeding (4%), bile leak (4%), pneumoperitoneum (3%), stent migration (2.7%), cholangitis (2.4%), abdominal pain (1.5%), and peritonitis (1.3%). Rare but serious adverse events included perforation (0.5%) and sepsis (0.3%). A single study within the analysis reported six procedure-related deaths, whereas none of the other included studies reported fatal complications.

When only procedures using transmural stent placement were analyzed, the overall rate of adverse events was 24.4% (114 of 467). The complications included stent migration (5.4%), pneumoperitoneum (3.4%), peritonitis (3%), hemorrhage (2.8%), cholangitis (3%), and bile leak (1.5%).[21]

With regard to the choice of intrahepatic or extrahepatic approach, both of the most recent meta-analyses indicate the extrahepatic approach is safer than intrahepatic approach. In the systematic review by Khan and colleagues,[26] transduodenal access had a pooled OR for adverse events of 0.4 (95% confidence interval, 0.18–0.87). Similarly, in the study by Wang and colleagues,[21] the pooled OR for the transduodenal approach was 0.61 (95% confidence interval, 0.36–1.03). A review comparing 211 extrahepatic and 138 intrahepatic drainage procedures found higher rates of adverse events when the intrahepatic approach was used (21.7% vs 9.9%; $P<.01$).[23] The higher rate of adverse events in the intrahepatic approach has been attributed to the longer distance of the tract through the liver parenchyma between the puncture site in the gastric wall and the intrahepatic bile duct, whereas the dilated common bile duct closely approximates the duodenal wall in the extrahepatic approach.

Adverse events are most closely linked to fistula dilation during EUS-BD. Sequential catheter dilations eliminates the need for cautery but may lead to separation of the liver and gastric wall, or between the duodenum and bile duct, because of forceful coaxial pushing. A balloon catheter can be used because it uses radial force rather than axial force, although the complication rate even when a balloon is used for dilation is similar to that seen with needle knife dilation.[21] These limitations may be addressed as improved specialized equipment for EUS-BD is developed and gains widespread use.

The meta-analysis comparing EUS-BD with PTBD in 483 patients found lower rates of severe complications, such as bile leaks, cholangitis, hemorrhage, or sepsis, in patients undergoing EUS-BD.[27] The rate of adverse events associated with PTBD is significant, as noted in a recent retrospective 10-year study of more than 2000 patients in which 40% experienced cholangitis, catheter malfunction, or displacement as either early or late complications.[28] These patients require reinterventions to maintain drainage, and cost-effectiveness seems to favor EUS-BD.

Nearly all of the published experience with EUS-BD is derived from expert centers with highly experienced therapeutic endoscopists. Thus, one cannot expect that these outcomes will be replicated as EUS-BD continues to grow in popularity. Maintaining safety and success requires the continued evolution of specialized tools for attaining biliary access and preventing complications, much in the way that a cautery-tipped delivery system has improved the speed and complexity of transmural drainage when compared with placement of multiple plastic stents. For instance, Park and colleagues[29] have described the use of a novel dedicated stent introducer for transmural BD that includes a fine tip and a metallic stent with anchoring flaps and an uncovered portion for anchoring within the intrahepatic ducts.

In cases of failed ERCP for BD, the endoscopist is thus left with several choices. We have seen from the existing data that in experienced hands EUS-BD is technically successful at the price of a high complication rate. The rate of severe adverse events for EUS-BD has been shown to actually be lower than that of PTBD, although it could be argued that revision of a malfunctioning percutaneous drain is more easily achieved without requiring an endoscopic procedure. Some experts obtain informed consent for EUS-BD even at the time of attempted ERCP, so that conversion in technique is achieved without the need for a second procedure. This is particularly appropriate if there is high suspicion for difficult ERCP, as in known duodenal obstruction or ampullary mass. For less experienced endoscopists, failure to achieve BD by ERCP should not automatically trigger an attempt at EUS-BD, because successful drainage may still be achieved by repeat ERCP at a tertiary center. Alternatively, despite its drawbacks, a percutaneous biliary drain may be an appropriate option based on the patient's underlying disease and local radiologic expertise.

THE CURRENT ROLE OF ENDOSCOPIC ULTRASOUND–GUIDED BILIARY DRAINAGE

Could EUS-BD replace ERCP as the primary therapy for biliary obstruction in selected cases? No robust data yet exists to compare the two approaches because nearly all of the accumulated data for EUS-BD have been from patients in whom ERCP was unsuccessful. However, Hara and colleagues[19] conducted a prospective study of EUS-CDS in 18 patients in whom EUS-BD was the primary therapy. In this study, technical and clinical success rate were both 94% with an 11% complication rate (peritonitis in two patients). This early success is encouraging, but was carried out in an expert center without any direct comparison with ERCP. A retrospective analysis comparing repeat ERCP with EUS-BD in cases of failed initial ERCP showed that both techniques were comparable in terms of successful stent placement (94.23% vs 93.26%) and adverse events (8.65% in both groups), with the risk of post-ERCP pancreatitis obviously lower in the EUS-BD group (4.8% vs 0%).[30] Advocates of EUS-BD cite the potential benefit of creating a new fistula via EUS-CDS or EUS-HGS in avoiding post-ERCP pancreatitis, because prolonged attempts at biliary cannulation are associated with a significantly increased risk of pancreatitis.

A single center retrospective study compared EUS-RV with needle knife papillotomy in patients with difficult cannulation of an accessible native papilla. In this study, EUS-RV was found to have a higher rate of technical success compared with needle knife papillotomy (98.3% vs 90.3%; $P = .03$) with similar complication rates (3.4% vs 6.9%; $P = .27$).[31] The design of the study called for a switch to either technique after five failed attempts with a guidewire and sphinterotome. Although the technical success of these procedures in expert hands is admirable, a mere five attempts at cannulation is a remarkably low threshold for abandoning traditional ERCP technique, particularly when the indication for the procedure is a nonmalignant condition, such as choledocholithaisis.

A recent international consensus statement access echoes the definition of difficult biliary cannulation as "the inability to achieve selective biliary cannulation by standard ERCP techniques within 10 minutes or up to 5 cannulation attempts or failure of access to the major papilla."[32] There is plenty of evidence demonstrating the increased incidence of post-ERCP pancreatitis with increased cannulation time, number of attempts, and number of pancreatic injections and cannulations.[33,34] However, alternative techniques, such as double-guidewire, pancreatic duct stent placement to facilitate biliary cannulation, and needle knife precut, may all be considered as techniques to improve the rate of cannulation. These techniques are familiar to any endoscopist with a high volume of ERCP procedures, and do not require the switch to EUS-BD with its attendant learning curve and complication rate. Until advances are made in the training and equipment for EUS-BD, such outcomes may be difficult to achieve outside of expert centers.

Given the limited number of patients and opportunities to use EUS-BD, mastery of all four techniques for intrahepatic and extrahepatic drainage may be difficult for providers in all but the highest-volume centers. The learning curve for EUS-HGS has been described by Oh and colleagues,[2] who noted a plateau of procedure time and adverse events after 33 cases. Given the infrequency of the need for these complex procedures, expertise may not develop rapidly. For example, in the prospective study to develop an anatomy-based algorithm for EUS-BD, only 52 patients were enrolled in a 4.5-year period.[10] Likewise, the enhanced-guidewire manipulation protocol described previously was studied over a 10-month period where the endoscopist performed 1350 ERCPs, with a mere 45 patients enrolled into the EUS-BD study because of failure of ERCP.[18] Tonozuka and colleagues[35] described their experience over a 12-month period in which 634 cases were performed: the papilla was inaccessible in 17 cases (2.7%) and ERCP failed in 11 cases (1.7%). EUS-BD was used in a total of 21 patients (3.3%), further illustrating the low number of opportunities to refine technique. To this end, Holt and colleagues[36] estimated that the total number of suitable EUS-BD cases per year in the United States lies somewhere between 1500 and 3500 cases nationwide, among a total of 500,000 ERCP procedures performed annually. Experience in these rare but complex procedures is thus best confined to a limited few until advances in training and equipment become more widespread.

An illustration of the difficulty in gaining expertise in EUS-BD is provided by the Spanish national survey where the technical success rate and adverse events of endoscopists performing less than 20 cases of EUS-guided biliary or pancreatic drainage were 67.2% and 23.2%, respectively.[37] Intraductal manipulation of the guidewire was found to be the most common factor in procedural failure, whereas most complications were linked to creation of the transmural fistula. In the retrospective comparison of repeat ERCP and EUS-BD by Dhir and colleagues,[30] both procedures were successful in placing a stent across the site of obstruction more than 90% of the time. Repeat ERCP thus remains a reasonable option even after an initial failed attempt if the papilla is accessible.

ENDOSCOPIC ULTRASOUND–GUIDED PANCREATIC DUCT DRAINAGE

The same principles used in EUS-BD can be used within the pancreatic duct when conventional ERP fails. The indications for EUS-guided pancreatic duct drainage (EUS-PDD) usually involve chronic pancreatitis or its sequelae, including main pancreatic duct stricture, duct leak, PD stones, or anastomotic stricture following pancreatic surgery. There are two options for performing EUS-PDD. The first is EUS-RV, where the pancreatic duct is accessed from the pancreatic body or tail (via transgastric approach) or the pancreatic head (via transduodenal approach). The pancreas is then punctured by a sharp 19-gauge needle and contrast is used to obtain a pancreatogram. An 0.035-inch or 0.025-inch stiff hydrophilic wire can then be advanced downstream into the lumen. Once the wire is coiled in position, RV proceeds in the typical manner. The second technique for EUS-PDD is transmural approach with fistula creation and AS. Following EUS-guided puncture into the pancreatic duct and placement of a wire, the needle tract can then be dilated by graded catheters, a low-profile balloon catheter, or cautery-assisted devices, such as a needle knife or cystotome. Following tract dilation, a stent is advanced into the pancreatic duct.

The stent may be placed across the papilla or pancreaticojejunal anastomosis, or it may be placed in a transluminal position at the access point gained by EUS. Both plastic stents and fully coated SEMS have been used for EUS-PDD.

The outcomes of EUS-PDD are described in retrospective series with generally small numbers of patients. A 2015 review including 222 patients reported a technical success rate of 77% and clinical success rate of 70% using either RV or AS. The complication rate was 19%, including abdominal pain (7.7%), acute pancreatitis (3.1%), bleeding (1.8%), perforation (0.9%), and isolated cases of pseudocyst and pneumoperitoneum.[38] A more recent international multicenter retrospective study of 80 patients described an improved technical success rate of 89%, immediate adverse events in 20% of patients, and delayed adverse events in 11%.[39]

Several barriers must be overcome to improve the outcomes of EUS-PDD and allow its expansion into wider use. The fibrotic pancreatic parenchyma may be difficult to traverse with needles or dilating devices, and aggressive attempts may result in procedure-related pancreatitis. An irregular duct with side branches may frustrate attempts to advance the guidewire, leading to shearing or wire perforation. The short length of the pancreatic duct may increase the risk of losing the position of the needle or wire.[40] The long-term outcomes are not well described, although it is disconcerting to note that 29% of the patients undergoing EUS-PDD in a 2007 series ultimately required surgery during a follow-up period of 4 to 36 months.[41] Finally, as in EUS-BD, there is a limited opportunity to perform these procedures to gain expertise, because ERP is generally successful when performed by experts in high-volume centers. Future directions will include prospective studies and improvement in technique with dedicated equipment.

SUMMARY

The current experience with EUS-BD shows that this therapeutic modality holds great promise but requires great skill and care. It is technically complex and difficult to learn, with limited opportunities outside of high-volume expert centers. Most practitioners of ERCP, particularly those with modest annual volumes of procedures, should not seek to add EUS-BD to their skill set at this time. Other options include a repeat attempt at ERCP on another day, referral to a tertiary center, or percutaneous BD. For those endoscopists who are already considered experts in ERCP, and have sufficient patient volume and complexity, EUS-BD may be an appropriate skill to learn.

Several things must be considered by the endoscopist considering use of EUS-BD. Informed consent for the ERCP procedure should include the risks and benefits of conversion to EUS-BD. The endoscopist should have appropriate surgical and interventional radiology support in case of failure or complications. There are two points of commitment during the procedure: the first is during contrast injection into the dilated biliary tree, because without completion of the drainage procedure the patient becomes at higher risk for cholangitis. The second point of commitment is during dilation of a tract if a new fistula is created for EUS-CDS or EUS-HGS. The dilation is the most critical step and associated with most of the complications for transmural stenting. Endoscopists gaining early experience may do well to follow published algorithms and master the extrahepatic approach or RV technique before learning the more difficult transluminal stent procedures.

As EUS-BD techniques are standardized and new equipment is developed to improve the speed, efficacy, and safety profile of these procedures, widespread adoption will become more feasible. High-volume expert centers will continue to refine techniques and collaborate to optimize equipment. In the meantime, lower-volume centers and community centers are better served by perfecting ERCP technique, because ERCP remains the highly successful standard for BD at the current time. Given the higher incidence of complications with EUS-BD, it is the endoscopist's responsibility to make certain that every available ERCP technique has been tried before even contemplating switching to EUS-BD, no matter the skill level of the endoscopist.

REFERENCES

1. Giovannini M, Moutardier V, Pesenti C, et al. Endoscopic ultrasound-guided bilio-duodenal anastomosis: a new technique for biliary drainage. Endoscopy 2001; 33(10):898–900.

2. Oh D, Park DH, Song TJ, et al. Optimal biliary access point and learning curve for endoscopic ultrasound-guided hepaticogastrostomy with transmural stenting. Therap Adv Gastroenterol 2017;10(1):42–53.

3. Park DH, Jang JW, Lee SS, et al. EUS-guided biliary drainage with transluminal stenting after failed ERCP: predictors of adverse events and long-term results. Gastrointest Endosc 2011;74(6):1276–84.

4. Umeda J, Itoi T, Tsuchiya T, et al. A newly designed plastic stent for EUS-guided hepaticogastrostomy: a prospective preliminary feasibility study (with videos). Gastrointest Endosc 2015;82(2):390–6.e2.

5. Nakai Y, Isayama H, Yamamoto N, et al. Safety and effectiveness of a long, partially covered metal stent for endoscopic ultrasound-guided hepaticogastrostomy in patients with malignant biliary obstruction. Endoscopy 2016;48(12): 1125–8.

6. Ogura T, Yamamoto K, Sano T, et al. Stent length is impact factor associated with stent patency in endoscopic ultrasound-guided hepaticogastrostomy. J Gastroenterol Hepatol 2015;30(12):1748–52.

7. Song TJ, Lee SS, Park DH, et al. Preliminary report on a new hybrid metal stent for EUS-guided biliary drainage (with videos). Gastrointest Endosc 2014;80(4): 707–11.

8. Paik WH, Park DH, Choi JH, et al. Simplified fistula dilation technique and modified stent deployment maneuver for EUS-guided hepaticogastrostomy. World J Gastroenterol 2014;20(17):5051–9.

9. Paik WH, Park DH. Endoscopic ultrasound-guided biliary access, with focus on technique and practical tips. Clin Endosc 2017;50(2):104–11.

10. Itoi T. Moving closer to developing an optimal algorithm for EUS-guided biliary drainage. Gastrointest Endosc 2016;84(6):947–9.

11. Ogura T, Higuchi K. Technical tips of endoscopic ultrasound-guided choledocho-duodenostomy. World J Gastroenterol 2015;21(3):820–8.

12. Perez-Miranda M, De la Serna Higuera C, Gil-Simon P, et al. EUS-guided chole-dochoduodenostomy with lumen-apposing metal stent after failed rendezvous in synchronous malignant biliary and gastric outlet obstruction (with video). Gastrointest Endosc 2014;80(2):342 [discussion: 343–4].

13. Kunda R, Pérez-Miranda M, Will U, et al. EUS-guided choledochoduodenostomy for malignant distal biliary obstruction using a lumen-apposing fully covered metal stent after failed ERCP. Surg Endosc 2016;30(11):5002–8.

14. Iwashita T, Yasuda I, Mukai T, et al. EUS-guided rendezvous for difficult biliary cannulation using a standardized algorithm: a multicenter prospective pilot study (with videos). Gastrointest Endosc 2016;83(2):394–400.

15. Savides TJ, Varadarajulu S, Palazzo L, EUS 2008 Working Group. EUS 2008 Working Group document: evaluation of EUS-guided hepaticogastrostomy. Gastrointest Endosc 2009;69(2 Suppl):S3–7.
16. Artifon EL, Marson FP, Gaidhane M, et al. Hepaticogastrostomy or choledocho-duodenostomy for distal malignant biliary obstruction after failed ERCP: is there any difference? Gastrointest Endosc 2015;81(4):950–9.
17. Tyberg A, Desai AP, Kumta NA, et al. EUS-guided biliary drainage after failed ERCP: a novel algorithm individualized based on patient anatomy. Gastrointest Endosc 2016;84(6):941–6.
18. Park DH, Jeong SU, Lee BU, et al. Prospective evaluation of a treatment algorithm with enhanced guidewire manipulation protocol for EUS-guided biliary drainage after failed ERCP (with video). Gastrointest Endosc 2013;78(1):91–101.
19. Hara K, Yamao K, Hijioka S, et al. Prospective clinical study of endoscopic ultrasound-guided choledochoduodenostomy with direct metallic stent placement using a forward-viewing echoendoscope. Endoscopy 2013;45(5):392–6.
20. Ikeuchi N, Itoi T. Endoscopic ultrasonography-guided biliary drainage: an alternative to percutaneous transhepatic puncture. Gastrointest Interv 2015;4:31–9.
21. Wang K, Zhu J, Xing L, et al. Assessment of efficacy and safety of EUS-guided biliary drainage: a systematic review. Gastrointest Endosc 2016;83(6):1218–27.
22. Dhir V, Bhandari S, Bapat M, et al. Comparison of transhepatic and extrahepatic routes for EUS-guided rendezvous procedure for distal CBD obstruction. United European Gastroenterol J 2013;1(2):103–8.
23. Dhir V, Artifon EL, Gupta K, et al. Multicenter study on endoscopic ultrasound-guided expandable biliary metal stent placement: choice of access route, direction of stent insertion, and drainage route. Dig Endosc 2014;26(3):430–5.
24. Kawakubo K, Isayama H, Kato H, et al. Multicenter retrospective study of endoscopic ultrasound-guided biliary drainage for malignant biliary obstruction in Japan. J Hepatobiliary Pancreat Sci 2014;21(5):328–34.
25. Poincloux L, Rouquette O, Buc E, et al. Endoscopic ultrasound-guided biliary drainage after failed ERCP: cumulative experience of 101 procedures at a single center. Endoscopy 2015;47(9):794–801.
26. Khan MA, Akbar A, Baron TH, et al. Endoscopic ultrasound-guided biliary drainage: a systematic review and meta-analysis. Dig Dis Sci 2016;61(3):684–703.
27. Sharaiha RZ, Khan MA, Kamal F, et al. Efficacy and safety of EUS-guided biliary drainage in comparison with percutaneous biliary drainage when ERCP fails: a systematic review and meta-analysis. Gastrointest Endosc 2017;85(5):904–14.
28. Nennstiel S, Weber A, Frick G, et al. Drainage-related complications in percutaneous transhepatic biliary drainage: an analysis over 10 years. J Clin Gastroenterol 2015;49(9):764–70.
29. Park DH, Lee TH, Paik WH, et al. Feasibility and safety of a novel dedicated device for one-step EUS-guided biliary drainage: a randomized trial. J Gastroenterol Hepatol 2015;30(10):1461–6.
30. Dhir V, Itoi T, Khashab MA, et al. Multicenter comparative evaluation of endoscopic placement of expandable metal stents for malignant distal common bile duct obstruction by ERCP or EUS-guided approach. Gastrointest Endosc 2015;81(4):913–23.
31. Dhir V, Bhandari S, Bapat M, et al. Comparison of EUS-guided rendezvous and precut papillotomy techniques for biliary access (with videos). Gastrointest Endosc 2012;75(2):354–9.

32. Liao WC, Angsuwatcharakon P, Isayama H, et al. International consensus recommendations for difficult biliary access. Gastrointest Endosc 2017;85(2):295–304.
33. Williams EJ, Taylor S, Fairclough P, et al. Risk factors for complication following ERCP; results of a large-scale, prospective multicenter study. Endoscopy 2007; 39(9):793–801.
34. Halttunen J, Meisner S, Aabakken L, et al. Difficult cannulation as defined by a prospective study of the Scandinavian Association for Digestive Endoscopy (SADE) in 907 ERCPs. Scand J Gastroenterol 2014;49(6):752–8.
35. Tonozuka R, Itoi T, Tsuchiya T, et al. EUS-guided biliary drainage is infrequently used even in high-volume centers of interventional EUS. Gastrointest Endosc 2016;84(1):206–7.
36. Holt BA, Hawes R, Hasan M. Biliary drainage: role of EUS guidance. Gastrointest Endosc 2016;83(1):160–5.
37. Vila JJ, Pérez-Miranda M, Vazquez-Sequeiros E, et al. Initial experience with EUS-guided cholangiopancreatography for biliary and pancreatic duct drainage: a Spanish national survey. Gastrointest Endosc 2012;76(6):1133–41.
38. Fujii-Lau LL, Levy MJ. Endoscopic ultrasound-guided pancreatic duct drainage. J Hepatobiliary Pancreat Sci 2015;22(1):51–7.
39. Tyberg A, Sharaiha RZ, Kedia P, et al. EUS-guided pancreatic drainage for pancreatic strictures after failed ERCP: a multicenter international collaborative study. Gastrointest Endosc 2017;85(1):164–9.
40. Devière J. EUS-guided pancreatic duct drainage: a rare indication in need of prospective evidence. Gastrointest Endosc 2017;85(1):178–80.
41. Will U, Fueldner F, Thieme AK, et al. Transgastric pancreatography and EUS-guided drainage of the pancreatic duct. J Hepatobiliary Pancreat Surg 2007; 14(4):377–82.

Endoscopic Ultrasound–Guided Gallbladder Drainage

Ryan Law, DO[a], Todd H. Baron, MD[b],*

KEYWORDS

- Cholecystitis • Lumen-apposing metal stents • EUS-guided gallbladder drainage
- Cholecystostomy

KEY POINTS

- Over the last decade, since first described, the techniques and indications for endoscopic ultrasound (EUS) -guided gallbladder drainage continue to evolve.
- Current data suggest that EUS-guided gallbladder intervention can be performed as primary therapy or secondary therapy in appropriate candidates.
- EUS-guided gallbladder drainage using a lumen-apposing metal stent can be performed for internalization of gallbladder drainage in patients with a percutaneous cholecystostomy catheter in situ and who are poor candidates for cholecystectomy.
- Following failed endoscopic retrograde cholangiopancreatography, EUS-guided gallbladder drainage can be performed to provide biliary decompression and a conduit for subsequent biliary rendezvous or antegrade therapy in patients with a patent cystic duct.

INTRODUCTION

The interventional capability of endoscopic ultrasound (EUS) has progressed considerably in recent years, most importantly in techniques for EUS-guided biliary drainage. EUS allows visualization of the intrahepatic and extrahepatic biliary tree, as well as the gallbladder, and provides a platform for various drainage techniques.[1,2] Technical interventions aimed at accessing the bile ducts and gallbladder continue to develop in parallel.

Conflicts of Interest/Disclosure: No conflicts of interest/disclosures (R. Law); W.L. Gore, Boston Scientific, Olympus, Cook Endoscopy (T.H. Baron).
Financial Support and Sponsorship: No financial support or sponsorship was required for construction of this article.
[a] Division of Gastroenterology, University of Michigan, 3912 Taubman Center, 1500 East Medical Center Drive, SPC 5362, Ann Arbor, MI 48109-5362, USA; [b] Division of Gastroenterology and Hepatology, University of North Carolina, 130 Mason Farm Road, CB 7080, Chapel Hill, NC 27599-0001, USA
* Corresponding author.
E-mail address: todd_baron@med.unc.edu

Gastrointest Endoscopy Clin N Am 28 (2018) 187–195
https://doi.org/10.1016/j.giec.2017.11.006
1052-5157/18/© 2017 Elsevier Inc. All rights reserved.

giendo.theclinics.com

Cholecystectomy persists as the standard of care for patients with acute calculous cholecystitis.[3] Some patients are poor surgical candidates because of significant medical comorbidities or prior abdominal surgery causing dense adhesions, or because of the sequelae of the cholecystitis itself, thus necessitating alternative interventions.[4,5] Historically, percutaneous cholecystostomy (PC) was performed for gallbladder decompression in these patients, either as destination therapy or as a bridge to subsequent cholecystectomy. Percutaneous drainage catheters require routine maintenance and catheter exchange and are often further limited by inadvertent dislodgement and patient discomfort.

In recent years, an alternative to PC has been developed that allows for internal drainage without many of the limitations of percutaneous drainage. EUS-guided transmural gallbladder was first described by Baron and Topazian in 2007[6] with the placement of a double-pigtail plastic stent for palliation of cholecystitis in a patient with unresectable hilar cholangiocarcinoma after failed attempts at endoscopic transpapillary gallbladder drainage. Since the initial description of EUS-guided transmural gallbladder drainage, substantial technical progress has been made, including placement of biliary fully covered self-expandable metal stents (FCSEMS) and the newer lumen-apposing metal stents (LAMS).

This article provides an update of recently published literature on the topic of EUS-guided gallbladder drainage. It should be noted that the use of stents for EUS-guided gallbladder drainage is not US Food and Drug Administration (FDA) approved and represents off-label use.

TECHNIQUE

- Monitored anesthesia care or endotracheal intubation is preferred for interventional EUS procedures.
- An oblique- or forward-viewing therapeutic curvilinear array echoendoscope is positioned in the duodenal bulb or distal gastric antrum to identify the gallbladder.
- A cursory diagnostic EUS examination should be completed to define the associated vascular anatomy adjacent to the intended needle path.
- The echoendoscope position is then stabilized, and a standard fine-needle aspiration (FNA) needle (most commonly 19 gauge) is used to puncture the gallbladder wall (**Fig. 1**).
- Accurate positioning can be confirmed by bile aspiration and/or cholecystography using water-soluble contrast medium.
- A standard 450-cm-long guidewire is then coiled within the gallbladder lumen (**Fig. 2**).
- The FNA needle is removed, and the tract is dilated using electrocautery (ie, cystotome, needle knife papillotome, or electrocautery-enhanced stent delivery system) or noncautery dilating device (ie, stepped axial dilators, dilating balloon).
- Following puncture and dilation, a stent (ie, double-pigtail plastic, FCSEMS, LAMS) is placed under endosonographic and fluoroscopic guidance.
- Although the technical placement of a double pigtail plastic stent and FCSEMS is widely understood, the placement of an LAMS is somewhat unique.
- After the LAMS delivery catheter is passed inside the gallbladder, the proximal flange of the stent is deployed under EUS guidance.
- The delivery system is then retracted slightly to create apposition.

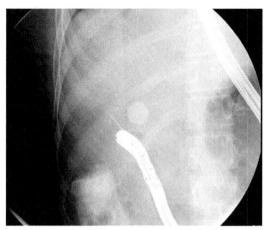

Fig. 1. Fluoroscopic image demonstrating identification of the gallbladder under endosonographic guidance with puncture of the gallbladder using a 19-g EUS-FNA needle.

- The distal flange can then be deployed under EUS guidance or endoscopic guidance with or without fluoroscopic guidance (discretion of the endoscopist) (**Fig. 3**).
- Following deployment of the distal flange, a double pigtail plastic stent is often placed within the LAMS for further stabilization and to prevent tissue overgrowth (**Fig. 4**).

An alternative to the above-mentioned steps is to proceed directly with placement of an LAMS with an electrocautery-enhanced delivery system. The puncture and deployment are done with one device. This approach is preferred by some endoscopists. The authors recommend that this approach be used by experts and when the gallbladder is markedly distended and the endoscope positioning is stable ("easy target"). They also recommend preloading the device with a guidewire for added safety. The wire is coiled within the gallbladder as soon as the delivery system enters the gallbladder lumen and before stent deployment.

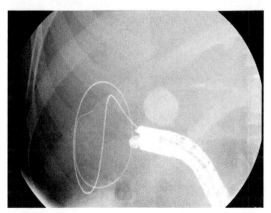

Fig. 2. Fluoroscopic image demonstrating passage of a long guidewire into the gallbladder lumen with creation of multiple loops to provide stable environment for subsequent stent placement.

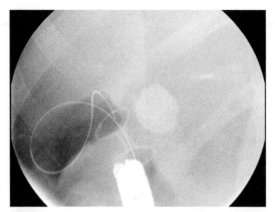

Fig. 3. Final fluoroscopic image following placement of an LAMS to create a cholecystoenterostomy.

OUTCOMES OF ENDOSCOPIC ULTRASOUND–GUIDED GALLBLADDER DRAINAGE

Endoscopic retrograde cholangiopancreatography (ERCP) with placement of a transpapillary plastic stent remains the standard method for endoscopic drainage of the gallbladder; however, EUS-guided transmural drainage from the adjacent gastrointestinal lumen has recently been developed because of inherent limitations of transpapillary stenting (ie, need for cystic duct patency, stent exchanges).[7]

Peñas-Herrero and colleagues[8] recently reviewed the published literature: 157 patients who underwent EUS-guided gallbladder drainage were identified. Studies using plastic stents, FCSEMS, and LAMS for transmural gallbladder drainage were included. Technical success was defined by successful stent deployment into the gallbladder

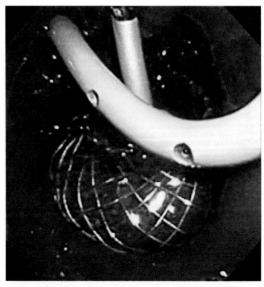

Fig. 4. Endoscopic image showing placement of a double pigtail plastic stent within the lumen of the LAMS to provide further stability and minimize the risk of tissue overgrowth if left in place long term.

and duodenum/stomach. Immediate clinical success was defined by resolution of acute cholecystitis. The overall technical and immediate clinical success was 97.5% and 99.3%, respectively, with technical failure occurring because of the inability to pass the guidewire, accidental guidewire loss, and stent misdeployment. Recurrent cholecystitis appears to be uncommon following successful stent placement and resolution of cholecystitis (≤3.5%), although long-term outcomes are less widely available. The overall aggregate adverse event rate from the included studies was 7.6%, with pneumoperitoneum being most common (6 patients). A similar systematic review by Anderloni and colleagues[9] demonstrated similar technical success, clinical success, and adverse event rates (96%, 93%, and 12%, respectively). Interestingly, the highest rate of adverse events occurred with plastic stent placement (18% vs 12% [FCSEMS] vs 10% [LAMS]). The earliest reports of EUS-guided gallbladder drainage described the use of double pigtail plastic stents for creation of the transmural tract; however, the small diameter of plastic stents makes them prone to clogging. EUS-guided gallbladder drainage evolved to the use of FCSEMS, and now to LAMS. Double pigtail plastic stents have largely fallen out of favor and are rarely used for this indication.

The recent availability of self-expandable LAMS has simplified EUS-guided gallbladder drainage.[2,10] The use of LAMS as primary therapy for poor operative candidates presenting with acute cholecystitis has been recently reviewed (**Fig. 5**).[11] Walter and colleagues[11] performed a prospective, multicenter study to determine efficacy and safety using EUS-guided gallbladder drainage using LAMS in 30 high-risk surgical candidates. Composite results yielded a technical success of 90% and clinical success of 96%, with a procedure- or stent-related adverse event rate of 13%. During a mean follow-up of 364 days, there were no episodes of stent migration. LAMS removal was performed in 50% of patients. In the remaining 15 patients, LAMS removal was not performed because of tissue overgrowth, patient refusal, and/or poor clinical condition. A second multicenter study by Irani and colleagues[12] included 15

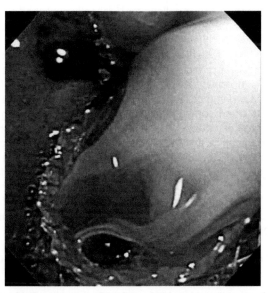

Fig. 5. Purulent drainage from the gallbladder following placement of an LAMS for the treatment of acute cholecystitis.

patients and demonstrated similar high technical and clinical success rates (93% and 100%, respectively) with an acceptable adverse event rate (7%). The recent FDA approval of an LAMS with an electrocautery-enhanced delivery catheter tip has further streamlined this procedure. This device minimizes accessory exchanges before stent placement and can be used without a guidewire in select patients (ie, "freehand" technique). A multicenter study including 75 patients who underwent EUS-guided gallbladder drainage with an electrocautery-enhanced LAMS has shown similar results.[13] Technical and clinical success was greater than 96% with an adverse event rate of 10%.

It should be noted that laparoscopic cholecystectomy may not be possible following EUS-guided gallbladder drainage with a LAMS because this procedure creates a permanent fistula between the gallbladder and adjacent gastrointestinal lumen. A prior study by Jang and colleagues[14] demonstrated successful laparoscopic cholecystectomy after EUS-guided gallbladder drainage; however, it should be noted that these patients were stented with 5-Fr nasobiliary tubes in comparison to the currently available 10-mm and 15-mm LAMS.

PERCUTANEOUS CHOLECYSTOSTOMY VERSUS ENDOSCOPIC ULTRASOUND–GUIDED TRANSMURAL GALLBLADDER DRAINAGE

As previously mentioned, PC remains the current standard of care for the treatment of acute cholecystitis in patients who are deemed inoperable with recent data suggesting increasing utilization. Duszak and Behrman[15] reported a nearly 10-fold increase in PC placement in the Medicare-age population from 2004 to 2009. However, PC catheters are uncomfortable, can dislodge, are often difficult to manage, and can adversely affect quality of life.[8] Furthermore, there remains up to a 41% risk of recurrent cholecystitis following PC catheter removal; thus, lifelong percutaneous drainage may be necessary in some patients, requiring routine catheter maintenance and catheter exchanges.[16]

Recent studies have aimed to compare outcomes of PC- and EUS-guided transmural gallbladder drainage. Irani and colleagues[17] recently published a multicenter, retrospective study to compare technical success, clinical success, and adverse events. There were no statistical differences in any measured parameter; however, there was a trend toward fewer adverse events in the EUS cohort. Statistical differences favoring the EUS-guided approach were noted when evaluating postprocedural pain (2.5 vs 6.5), length of hospital stay (3 days vs 9 days), and number of repeat interventions (11 vs 112). Tyberg and colleagues[18] also identified an increase in the number of repeat interventions when comparing PC- and EUS-guided drainage (24% vs 10%; $P = .037$). No differences in technical success, clinical success, or adverse events were noted. An additional 1:1 matched cohort study by Teoh and colleagues[19] also comparing PC- and EUS-guided transmural gallbladder drainage in 118 patients (59 patients in each cohort) support the above data. Similar rates for technical and clinical success were identified, but a statistical difference was noted in adverse events (32% vs 75%) and severe adverse events (24% vs 75%) favoring the EUS approach. A trend toward clinical significance favoring the EUS approach was also seen regarding recurrent cholecystitis (0% vs 7%).

ALTERNATE INDICATIONS FOR ENDOSCOPIC ULTRASOUND–GUIDED GALLBLADDER DRAINAGE

In addition to primary gallbladder drainage for cholecystitis, EUS-guided LAMS can also be placed to internalize biliary drainage in poor surgical candidates with acute cholecystitis who have indwelling percutaneous drains.[20] The authors recently published data on 7 such patients and noted an immediate technical success of 100% with no immediate or delayed adverse events, and no recurrence of acute cholecystitis or need for surgical intervention after percutaneous catheter removal.

Following EUS-guided gallbladder drainage, the tract can subsequently be used as a conduit for further biliary interventions. Ge and colleagues[21] reported a small case series (n = 7) describing EUS-guided gallbladder drainage using an LAMS and subsequent cholecystoscopy with removal of gallstones, and gallbladder polypectomy. A similar study by Chan and colleagues[22] also described cholecystoscopy after EUS-guided gallbladder drainage using an LAMS in a small cohort of patients (n = 25). The cholecystoenteric fistula permitted stone retrieval, laser lithotripsy, and a variety of advanced imaging modalities (ie, magnification endoscopy, miniprobe EUS, endocytoscopy, confocal endomicroscopy).

The authors recently published a report of a medically complicated patient who presented with cholangitis and cholecystitis that underwent EUS-guided gallbladder drainage following failed ERCP due to an intradiverticular papilla.[23] Gallbladder drainage was performed to treat acute cholecystitis; however, the cholecystoenterostomy was subsequently used to perform a biliary rendezvous procedure facilitating ERCP with sphincterotomy and stone clearance.

Finally, EUS-guided gallbladder drainage can be used for palliation of malignant distal biliary obstruction when ERCP fails and EUS-guided biliary drainage (ie, choledochoduodenostomy or hepaticogastrostomy) is unsuccessful or impractical.[24] Although this technique can be considered in such circumstances, it should be noted that cystic duct patency is mandatory to provide palliative drainage.

SUMMARY

In conclusion, EUS-guided gallbladder drainage is an effective and safe treatment option in patients with poor surgical candidacy who present with acute cholecystitis. This procedure may serve as destination therapy or as a bridge to future surgical intervention. Although acute cholecystitis remains the main indication for this procedure, additional clinical scenarios have been described whereby this technique may be useful. Technical improvements and device innovation, namely LAMS, have streamlined the procedure; however, expert-level endoscopic skill remains a necessity. Further study of EUS-guided gallbladder drainage techniques will be essential to determining optimal treatment algorithms and in resolving the remaining technical challenges of this procedure.

REFERENCES

1. Poincloux L, Rouquette O, Buc E, et al. Endoscopic ultrasound-guided biliary drainage after failed ERCP: cumulative experience of 101 procedures at a single center. Endoscopy 2015;47:794–801.
2. de la Serna-Higuera C, Perez-Miranda M, Gil-Simon P, et al. EUS-guided transenteric gallbladder drainage with a new fistula-forming, lumen-apposing metal stent. Gastrointest Endosc 2013;77:303–8.
3. Baron TH, Grimm IS, Swanstrom LL. Interventional approaches to gallbladder disease. N Engl J Med 2015;373:357–65.
4. Karakayali FY, Akdur A, Kirnap M, et al. Emergency cholecystectomy vs percutaneous cholecystostomy plus delayed cholecystectomy for patients with acute cholecystitis. Hepatobiliary Pancreat Dis Int 2014;13:316–22.

5. Simorov A, Ranade A, Parcells J, et al. Emergent cholecystostomy is superior to open cholecystectomy in extremely ill patients with acalculous cholecystitis: a large multicenter outcome study. Am J Surg 2013;206:935–40 [discussion: 40–1].

6. Baron TH, Topazian MD. Endoscopic transduodenal drainage of the gallbladder: implications for endoluminal treatment of gallbladder disease. Gastrointest Endosc 2007;65:735–7.

7. Itoi T, Coelho-Prabhu N, Baron TH. Endoscopic gallbladder drainage for management of acute cholecystitis. Gastrointest Endosc 2010;71:1038–45.

8. Peñas-Herrero I, de la Serna-Higuera C, Perez-Miranda M. Endoscopic ultrasound-guided gallbladder drainage for the management of acute cholecystitis (with video). J Hepatobiliary Pancreat Sci 2015;22:35–43.

9. Anderloni A, Buda A, Vieceli F, et al. Endoscopic ultrasound-guided transmural stenting for gallbladder drainage in high-risk patients with acute cholecystitis: a systematic review and pooled analysis. Surg Endosc 2016;30:5200–8.

10. Moon JH, Choi HJ, Kim DC, et al. A newly designed fully covered metal stent for lumen apposition in EUS-guided drainage and access: a feasibility study (with videos). Gastrointest Endosc 2014;79:990–5.

11. Walter D, Teoh AY, Itoi T, et al. EUS-guided gall bladder drainage with a lumen-apposing metal stent: a prospective long-term evaluation. Gut 2016;65:6–8.

12. Irani S, Baron TH, Grimm IS, et al. EUS-guided gallbladder drainage with a lumen-apposing metal stent (with video). Gastrointest Endosc 2015;82:1110–5.

13. Dollhopf M, Larghi A, Will U, et al. EUS-guided gallbladder drainage in patients with acute cholecystitis and high surgical risk using an electrocautery-enhanced lumen-apposing metal stent device. Gastrointest Endosc 2017;86: 636–43.

14. Jang JW, Lee SS, Song TJ, et al. Endoscopic ultrasound-guided transmural and percutaneous transhepatic gallbladder drainage are comparable for acute cholecystitis. Gastroenterology 2012;142:805–11.

15. Duszak R Jr, Behrman SW. National trends in percutaneous cholecystostomy between 1994 and 2009: perspectives from Medicare provider claims. J Am Coll Radiol 2012;9:474–9.

16. McKay A, Abulfaraj M, Lipschitz J. Short- and long-term outcomes following percutaneous cholecystostomy for acute cholecystitis in high-risk patients. Surg Endosc 2012;26:1343–51.

17. Irani S, Ngamruengphong S, Teoh A, et al. Similar efficacies of endoscopic ultrasound gallbladder drainage with a lumen-apposing metal stent versus percutaneous transhepatic gallbladder drainage for acute cholecystitis. Clin Gastroenterol Hepatol 2017;15:738–45.

18. Tyberg A, Saumoy M, Sequeiros EV, et al. EUS-guided versus percutaneous gallbladder drainage: isn't it time to convert? J Clin Gastroenterol 2018;52:79–84.

19. Teoh AYB, Serna C, Penas I, et al. Endoscopic ultrasound-guided gallbladder drainage reduces adverse events compared with percutaneous cholecystostomy in patients who are unfit for cholecystectomy. Endoscopy 2017;49:130–8.

20. Law R, Grimm IS, Stavas JM, et al. Conversion of percutaneous cholecystostomy to internal transmural gallbladder drainage using an endoscopic ultrasound-guided, lumen-apposing metal stent. Clin Gastroenterol Hepatol 2016;14:476–80.

21. Ge N, Sun S, Sun S, et al. Endoscopic ultrasound-assisted transmural cholecystoduodenostomy or cholecystogastrostomy as a bridge for per-oral cholecystoscopy therapy using double-flanged fully covered metal stent. BMC Gastroenterol 2016; 16:9.

22. Chan SM, Teoh AYB, Yip HC, et al. Feasibility of per-oral cholecystoscopy and advanced gallbladder interventions after EUS-guided gallbladder stenting (with video). Gastrointest Endosc 2017;85:1225–32.
23. Law R, Baron TH. Endoscopic ultrasound-guided gallbladder drainage to facilitate biliary rendezvous for the management of cholangitis due to choledocholithiasis. Endoscopy 2017;49:E309–10.
24. Imai H, Kitano M, Omoto S, et al. EUS-guided gallbladder drainage for rescue treatment of malignant distal biliary obstruction after unsuccessful ERCP. Gastrointest Endosc 2016;84:147–51.

Novel Uses of Lumen-Apposing Metal Stents

Monica Saumoy, MD, MS[a], Clark Yarber[b], Michel Kahaleh, MD[a],*

KEYWORDS

- LAMS • Endoscopic gastrojejunostomy • Endoscopic

KEY POINTS

- The lumen apposing metal stent (LAMS) can be used in any scenario that would benefit from creation of an anastomosis, such as drainage, relief from gastric outlet obstruction, or creating a fistulous tract for further endoscopic intervention.
- These novel uses of the LAMS provide a minimally invasive alternative for various procedures for patients, forgoing the risk of surgery, which decreases hospital stay and improves quality of life.
- Common limitations of the LAMS include migration, intolerance of the stents, and inability to approximate the 2 desired apposed lumens.
- In the future, the creation of longer, as well as wider, stents may facilitate the use of the LAMS for a wider range of procedures.

INTRODUCTION

The lumen apposing metal stent (LAMS) has been well described for drainage of pancreatic fluid collections.[1] The unique dog bone, or yoyo, design maintains a stable anastomosis to allow for direct apposition of the 2 separate lumens. By creating a stable conduit using a fully covered stent, a LAMS decreases the risk of leakage of enteric contents. The large stent diameter gives an enhanced access point for drainage, decreasing the risk of obstruction with intestinal material. In addition, an endoscope can enter the bridged lumen through the stent to allow for endoscopic manipulation. Other well-described indications for LAMS include bile duct drainage for choledocho-duodenostomy and endoscopic gallbladder drainage.[2,3] In addition to the tightly sealed apposition between the 2 surfaces, the fully covered design of the stent allows removal when the fistulous tract is no longer needed.

Disclosure: Dr M. Kahaleh receives grant support from Boston Scientific. Drs M. Saumoy and C. Yarber have no disclosures.
[a] Division of Gastroenterology and Hepatology, Weill Cornell Medicine, New York Presbyterian Hospital, 1305 York Avenue, 4th Floor, New York, NY 10021, USA; [b] Central Michigan University, College of Medicine, Mount Pleasant, MI 48859, USA
* Corresponding author.
E-mail address: mkahaleh@gmail.com

More recently, novel indications for the LAMS have been continuously developed by taking advantage of the stent shape. For example, in patients with altered anatomy such as Billroth II or Roux-en-Y gastric bypass, fistula creation can facilitate other therapeutic procedures. This is with creation of a jejunojejunostomy or gastrogastric fistula as part of the endoscopic ultrasound (EUS)-directed transgastric endoscopic retrograde cholangiopancreatography (ERCP) (EDGE). A LAMS can also be used to manage surgical complications, such as enlargement of a surgical anastomosis or drainage of a surgical collection, such as biloma. Additionally, endoscopic gastrojejunostomy (GJ) has been developed for management of gastric outlet obstruction (GOO). Finally, a LAMS can be used for drainage of any other parenteral abscess cavity. These novel indications for a LAMS further demonstrate that the applications for this stent are potentially limitless in situations that require the creation of a stable fistulous tract.

ALTERNATIVE DRAINAGE ACCESS

The use of LAMS for EUS-guided abscess drainage emerged as an alternative to other minimally invasive, percutaneous techniques. Traditionally, drainage of pancreatic fluid collections was performed transgastrically. However, creation of a fistula for drainage into an infected cavity can be performed in any part of the accessible intestinal tract. Previously, computed tomography–guided and ultrasound–guided drainage of abscesses have been the most clinically accepted methods for drainage. However, percutaneous catheters have limitations. For example, with percutaneous drainage, passing through other organs is often unavoidable. When the percutaneous drain is in place, patients complain of the morbidity associated with having an external drain, which can become dislodged and require additional procedures.[4,5] EUS-guided drainage does not have these limitations, and abscesses often lie in close proximity to the gastrointestinal (GI) tract. Therefore, endoscopically preformed drainage has become an exciting alternative.

Rodrigues-Pinto and Baron[6] demonstrated a novel use of a EUS-guided LAMS for drainage of an infected aortic aneurysmal sac after endovascular stent graft placement for thoracoabdominal aortic aneurysm. Given the location, the abscess was not accessible percutaneously. After deployment, the patient improved with resolution of the abscess after 48 hours. In addition to an alternative site for abscess drainage from the upper GI tract, Poincloux and colleagues[4] demonstrated the use of the LAMS for EUS-guided drainage of pelvic abscesses. Under fluoroscopic and EUS guidance, fistula was created between the colon or rectum and the cavity of the abscess. In their case series of 37 subjects, only 4 underwent drainage with a LAMS. Two subjects had successful EUS-guided drainage with a LAMS, whereas the other 2 subjects experienced complications. One subject had diverticulitis complicated by an abscess and, after undergoing a transcolonic LAMS procedure, the subject developed pain, sepsis, and subsequently required surgical exploration that revealed perforation of the infected diverticulum. That subject had multiple risk factors (long-term steroids and chronic inflammatory disease) that may have led to this complication. The second subject who underwent transrectal abscess drainage with a LAMS secondary to an abscess related to uterine cancer had recurrence of the abscess at 3 months. Though current small case series suggest that drainage of diverticular abscesses may have lower treatment success compared with other abscess causes, additional improvements in methods can further improve the clinical success rates.[7,8]

Despite these cases of a small number of subjects, EUS-guided drainage of thoracic or pelvic abscess can be a potential alternative to surgical and percutaneous interventions. Future studies will further elucidate the potential of LAMS use with abscess cavity drainage.

BENIGN INTESTINAL STRICTURES

Benign GI strictures are typically managed with endoscopic balloon dilation (EBD) because of its positive short-term results.[9] However, EBD treatment of strictures is limited by its high recurrence rate and requires multiple sessions.[9] Therefore, clinicians have turned toward LAMS use as a potential alternative to maintain the patency of the intestinal lumen (**Fig. 1**).

Irani and colleagues[10] retrospectively studied 25 subjects who underwent LAMS placement for benign GI strictures. The strictures in these cases were throughout the GI tract, including postesophagectomy strictures, gastric bypass strictures, pyloric stenosis, and so forth. The purpose of this study arose out of the need for a stent with a lower migration rate in GI strictures when compared with a fully covered self-expanding metal stent (FCSEMS) or a plastic stent, which have demonstrated migration rates of up to 30% to 40%.[11,12] Clinical success was defined by resolution of symptoms at least 6 months after stent placement, which was achieved in 60% of the subjects. The migration rate in the study was 7%, which compares favorably with an FCSEMS secured with over-the-scope clips (15%) or sutures (up to 33%).[13,14]

Another case series by Majumder and colleagues[9] described using a LAMS for benign esophageal strictures. Three subjects underwent successful esophageal stricture dilation with a LAMS after unsuccessful EBD. The investigators listed potential reasons for success, such as the lack of need for multiple repeated procedures and the lower risk for perforation, mitigated by the fully covered design of the stents. This contrasts with endoscopic dilation, which may require several procedures and carries an increased risk of perforation.[15–20]

Similar to esophageal strictures, pyloric stenosis has a similar need for retreatment after EBD in benign disease.[21,22] French and colleagues[23] used the LAMS in 10 subjects with pyloric stenosis, with a 90% clinical success rate. One-half of the subjects had previously failed EBD. In this case series, the LAMS was well tolerated and did not migrate, which is in contrast to the 63% migration rate for the FCSEMS in benign pyloric strictures.[24] The success and, particularly, the lack of migration are attributed to the unique design of the LAMS.

The novel use of the LAMS in benign intestinal strictures has shown a positive safety profile and low migration rate. However, management of benign strictures with a

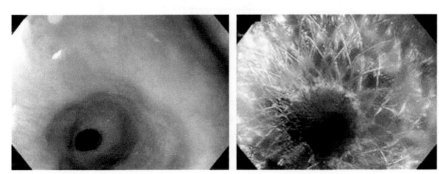

Fig. 1. Endoscopic view of a LAMS deployed across the esophagus for benign stricture.

LAMS remains a novel therapeutic method and larger studies prospectively comparing the LAMS with the FCSEMS with EBD are still necessary.

ALTERED ANATOMY

Patients with pancreaticobiliary diseases and altered anatomy were previously only able to be successfully managed either surgically (laparoscopic assisted), or percutaneously. Alternatively, deep enteroscopy-assisted ERCP has a success rate of 63%, which depends on the length of the roux limb.[25,26] However, with the development of the LAMS, patients with altered anatomy can undergo fistula creation to facilitate additional therapeutic procedures.

Kedia and colleagues[27] described the creation of a gastrogastric fistula as part of the EDGE procedure in 5 subjects with Roux-en-Y bypass for management of pancreaticobiliary disorders. (**Fig. 2**) EUS-guided placement of a LAMS for creation of a fistula between the gastric remnant and the excluded stomach was successful in 100% of cases. Subsequent ERCP was successful in only 3 of 5 cases due to the inability to pass the duodenoscope through the newly created fistula. To avoid the risk of stent dislodgement in these 2 subjects, ERCP was postponed. The LAMS was left in place for at least 3 weeks, after which these subjects had a follow-up ERCP with LAMS removal and closure of the fistula. Stent dislodgement was the only complication associated with EDGE in this series. The investigators comment that this technique can be complicated by LAMS migration, causing peritonitis and potential weight regain on creation of the fistula. With the future development of a larger diameter LAMS, the rates of stent dislodgement will decrease to allow for ease of passage of the duodenoscope.

Billroth II anatomy has also been successfully managed with LAMS. A case series by Rodrigues-Pinto and colleagues[28] described management of afferent limb syndrome in 4 subjects with Billroth II reconstruction. EUS-guided creation of an anastomosis using LAMS can bypass the obstructed afferent limb as a more durable treatment option than repeated EBD and forgoes the risk of surgical intervention. This particular case series involved the creation of jejunojejunostomy,

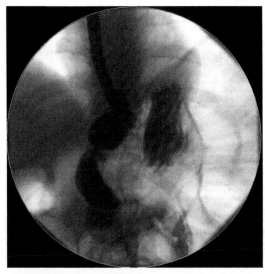

Fig. 2. Contrast evaluation of gastrogastric fistula for EDGE.

gastrojejunostomy, or duodenojejunostomy. However, the duration of stent placement to prevent recurrences of afferent limb syndrome remains unknown. In the case series, the only complication was seen in 1 subject who had the stent removed, resulting in closure of the anastomosis and recurrence of afferent limb syndrome. Long-term studies are required to determine the duration of stent placement that will lead to a permanent patent fistula after stent removal. The long-term effects of stent placement must also be studied because these stents are not intended for permanent use.

The use of the LAMS in patients with altered anatomy, for jejunojejunostomy in afferent limb syndrome, or gastrogastric fistula for EDGE is a novel intervention that subverts the need for surgery. As previously mentioned, limitations of these novel therapeutic procedures with LAMS further emphasize the need for larger, longer term studies to determine the safety and consequences of creating these anastomoses. However, given the data that are currently available combined with technological advances in stent design, there is reason for optimism that these minimally invasive interventions could someday become mainstream.

THE LUMEN APPOSING METAL STENT FOR SUTURE-LESS GASTROJEJUNOSTOMY

The use of the LAMS for EUS-GJ was born from the need for a durable alternative for palliation of malignant GOO (**Fig. 3**). Endoscopic management with enteral stenting was initially limited by the high rates of reintervention. Placement of these enteral stents had high success rates with a rapid time to resumption of food as compared with surgical GJ.[29] However, these metal stents were complicated by tumor ingrowth, stent migration, food impaction, and stent collapse.[21] Therefore, enteral stenting was primarily used to improve quality of life in patients with a short life expectancy. Surgical GJ is a durable alternative; however, many patients are considered poor surgical candidates given the underlying malnutrition, advanced malignancy, and short life expectancy.[30] And given the high morbidity of surgical GJ, reported as high as 39%, this technique has a limited role to palliate patients with malignant GOO.[31]

GJ (or gastroduodenostomy, depending on which target organ is closer and if the duodenum is not obstructed by tumor involvement) is performed using the 15 mm

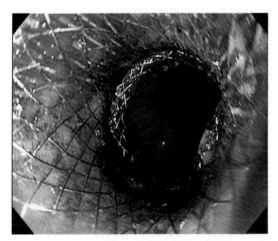

Fig. 3. Contrast evaluation of GJ in patient with malignant GOO.

LAMS to take advantage of the largest diameter stent lumen to prevent stent obstruction. Currently, there are multiple techniques that have been described to identify a suitable loop of small intestine to create the anastomosis.[32] The 5 techniques are (1) antegrade EUS-gastroenterostomy (EUS-GE), the traditional method; (2) antegrade EUS-GE, the rendezvous method; (3) retrograde EUS-GE, enterogastrostomy, (4) EUS–double-balloon-occluded gastrojejunostomy bypass (EPASS); and (5) antegrade EUS-GJ, the direct method.

In a retrospective study by Khashab and colleagues,[33] 10 subjects underwent EUS-GJ. Three of the subjects had malignant GOO and 1 had a complete obstruction requiring direct EUS-GJ. The other 9 subjects underwent balloon-assisted EUS-GJ, 8 of which were successful. Therefore, the technical success of this study was 90%. Losing position of the guidewire and pushing the small bowel distally are 2 challenges commonly encountered with EUS-GJ. Clinical success was achieved in all 9 subjects who underwent successful EUS-GJ, defined by subject's ability to tolerate oral intake. No symptom recurrence was found at a mean follow-up of 150 days and there were no adverse events.

A prospective study by Itoi and colleagues[34] evaluated the use of EPASS using a LAMS. This study included 20 subjects with malignant GOO. The investigators reported a technical success rate of 90% (18 out of 20). Two of the cases were complicated by advancing the guidewire and pushing the distending jejunum distally, leading to misdeployment of the LAMS, resulting in pneumoperitoneum. A large diameter guidewire or an overtube was used to avoid the looping of the balloon tube in the stomach. The cautery-assisted LAMS simplified the procedure and avoided the need for tract dilation.

A retrospective study by Tyberg and colleagues[35] described 26 subjects with GOO who underwent EUS-GJ with a LAMS. Subjects with both benign and malignant GOO were included in this study. Technical success was achieved in 24 subjects (92%). Clinical success was achieved in 22 subjects (85%). Cautery-assisted LAMS was used in 9 subjects. Stent misdeployment occurred in 27% of subjects, who were successfully bridged with an FCSEMS. However, 3 of the subjects had complications, including peritonitis, bleeding, and abdominal pain resulting in surgery.

The high technical and clinical success rates of these studies indicate that EUS-GJ is a promising novel technique for GOO. Based on these small case series, long-term efficacy is suggested to be similar to that seen in surgical GJ. The development of a more advanced delivery system, and larger diameter LAMS would also mitigate many of the technical difficulties for this procedure.

THE LUMEN APPOSING METAL STENT FOR BARIATRIC INDICATIONS

Current case studies demonstrate the use of LAMS after surgical complications of bariatric surgery. However, future uses for bariatric purposes may include suturing the pylorus, effectively causing a GOO, and subsequently creating a bypass fistula using a LAMS to form the anastomosis. This would theoretically function similarly to a Roux-en-Y bypass, but techniques are still being developed for this purpose.

SUMMARY

The novel use of the LAMS will continue to develop throughout the next decade as future endoscopists take advantage of the anticipated future improvement in the design of the LAMS.

The unique design of LAMS decreases the migration rate and improves patient tolerance. Long-term data must be collected and analyzed to determine the long-term efficacy for these novel indications of LAMS. Additionally, future studies are necessary to determine potential risks of leaving the stents in place for extended periods of time. As more designs of LAMS are produced to increase the length and diameter of the stents, the range of procedural interventions that can be performed will continue to broaden. Theoretically, this will reduce the need for surgical and percutaneous interventions. The studies outlined in this article article show promising results for the novel uses of the LAMS, and such interventions are revolutionizing the landscape of interventional endoscopy.

REFERENCES

1. Siddiqui AA, Adler DG, Nieto J, et al. EUS-guided drainage of peripancreatic fluid collections and necrosis by using a novel lumen-apposing stent: a large retrospective, multicenter U.S. experience (with videos). Gastrointest Endosc 2016; 83(4):699–707.
2. Irani S, Ngamruengphong S, Teoh A, et al. Similar efficacies of endoscopic ultrasound gallbladder drainage with a lumen-apposing metal stent versus percutaneous transhepatic gallbladder drainage for acute cholecystitis. Clin Gastroenterol Hepatol 2017;15(5):738–45.
3. Kunda R, Perez-Miranda M, Will U, et al. EUS-guided choledochoduodenostomy for malignant distal biliary obstruction using a lumen-apposing fully covered metal stent after failed ERCP. Surg Endosc 2016;30(11):5002–8.
4. Poincloux L, Caillol F, Allimant C, et al. Long-term outcome of endoscopic ultrasound-guided pelvic abscess drainage: a two-center series. Endoscopy 2017;49(5):484–90.
5. McGahan JP, Lindfors KK. Percutaneous cholecystostomy: an alternative to surgical cholecystostomy for acute cholecystitis? Radiology 1989;173(2):481–5.
6. Rodrigues-Pinto E, Baron TH. Endoscopic ultrasound-guided transesophageal drainage of an infected aneurysm after aortic stent graft placement. Gastroenterology 2016;151(1):30–1.
7. Ramesh J, Bang JY, Trevino J, et al. Comparison of outcomes between endoscopic ultrasound-guided transcolonic and transrectal drainage of abdominopelvic abscesses. J Gastroenterol Hepatol 2013;28(4):620–5.
8. Puri R, Choudhary NS, Kotecha H, et al. Endoscopic ultrasound-guided pelvic and prostatic abscess drainage: experience in 30 patients. Indian J Gastroenterol 2014;33(5):410–3.
9. Majumder S, Buttar NS, Gostout C, et al. Lumen-apposing covered self-expanding metal stent for management of benign gastrointestinal strictures. Endosc Int Open 2016;4(1):E96–101.
10. Irani S, Jalaj S, Ross A, et al. Use of a lumen-apposing metal stent to treat GI strictures (with videos). Gastrointest Endosc 2017;85(6):1285–9.
11. Hirdes MM, Siersema PD, Vleggaar FP. A new fully covered metal stent for the treatment of benign and malignant dysphagia: a prospective follow-up study. Gastrointest Endosc 2012;75(4):712–8.
12. Ham YH, Kim GH. Plastic and biodegradable stents for complex and refractory benign esophageal strictures. Clin Endosc 2014;47(4):295–300.
13. Irani S, Baron TH, Gluck M, et al. Preventing migration of fully covered esophageal stents with an over-the-scope clip device (with videos). Gastrointest Endosc 2014;79(5):844–51.

14. Fujii LL, Bonin EA, Baron TH, et al. Utility of an endoscopic suturing system for prevention of covered luminal stent migration in the upper GI tract. Gastrointest Endosc 2013;78(5):787–93.

15. Silvis SE, Nebel O, Rogers G, et al. Endoscopic complications. Results of the 1974 American Society for Gastrointestinal Endoscopy Survey. JAMA 1976; 235(9):928–30.

16. Piotet E, Escher A, Monnier P. Esophageal and pharyngeal strictures: report on 1,862 endoscopic dilatations using the Savary-Gilliard technique. Eur Arch Otorhinolaryngol 2008;265(3):357–64.

17. Pereira-Lima JC, Ramires RP, Zamin I Jr, et al. Endoscopic dilation of benign esophageal strictures: report on 1043 procedures. Am J Gastroenterol 1999; 94(6):1497–501.

18. Mandelstam P, Sugawa C, Silvis SE, et al. Complications associated with esophagogastroduodenoscopy and with esophageal dilation. Gastrointest Endosc 1976;23(1):16–9.

19. Karnak I, Tanyel FC, Buyukpamukcu N, et al. Esophageal perforations encountered during the dilation of caustic esophageal strictures. J Cardiovasc Surg (Torino) 1998;39(3):373–7.

20. Hernandez LV, Jacobson JW, Harris MS. Comparison among the perforation rates of Maloney, balloon, and savary dilation of esophageal strictures. Gastrointest Endosc 2000;51(4 Pt 1):460–2.

21. Brimhall B, Adler DG. Enteral stents for malignant gastric outlet obstruction. Gastrointest Endosc Clin N Am 2011;21(3):389–403, vii-viii.

22. Lau JY, Chung SC, Sung JJ, et al. Through-the-scope balloon dilation for pyloric stenosis: long-term results. Gastrointest Endosc 1996;43(2 Pt 1):98–101.

23. French PC, Holmsen H, Stormorken H. Adenine nucleotide metabolism of blood platelets. VII. ATPases: subcellular localization and behaviour during the thrombin-platelet interaction. Biochim Biophys Acta 1970;206(3):438–48.

24. Choi WJ, Park JJ, Park J, et al. Effects of the temporary placement of a self-expandable metallic stent in benign pyloric stenosis. Gut Liver 2013;7(4):417–22.

25. Shah RJ, Smolkin M, Yen R, et al. A multicenter, U.S. experience of single-balloon, double-balloon, and rotational overtube-assisted enteroscopy ERCP in patients with surgically altered pancreaticobiliary anatomy (with video). Gastrointest Endosc 2013;77(4):593–600.

26. Schreiner MA, Chang L, Gluck M, et al. Laparoscopy-assisted versus balloon enteroscopy-assisted ERCP in bariatric post-Roux-en-Y gastric bypass patients. Gastrointest Endosc 2012;75(4):748–56.

27. Kedia P, Tyberg A, Kumta NA, et al. EUS-directed transgastric ERCP for Roux-en-Y gastric bypass anatomy: a minimally invasive approach. Gastrointest Endosc 2015;82(3):560–5.

28. Rodrigues-Pinto E, Grimm IS, Baron TH. Efficacy of endoscopically created bypass anastomosis in treatment of afferent limb syndrome: a single-center study. Clin Gastroenterol Hepatol 2016;14(4):633–7.

29. Maetani I, Tada T, Ukita T, et al. Comparison of duodenal stent placement with surgical gastrojejunostomy for palliation in patients with duodenal obstructions caused by pancreaticobiliary malignancies. Endoscopy 2004;36(1):73–8.

30. Frech EJ, Adler DG. Endoscopic therapy for malignant bowel obstruction. J Support Oncol 2007;5(7):303–10, 319.

31. Medina-Franco H, Abarca-Perez L, Espana-Gomez N, et al. Morbidity-associated factors after gastrojejunostomy for malignant gastric outlet obstruction. Am Surg 2007;73(9):871–5.

32. Irani S, Baron TH, Itoi T, et al. Endoscopic gastroenterostomy: techniques and re-view. Curr Opin Gastroenterol 2017;33(5):320–9.
33. Khashab MA, Kumbhari V, Grimm IS, et al. EUS-guided gastroenterostomy: the first U.S. clinical experience (with video). Gastrointest Endosc 2015;82(5):932–8.
34. Itoi T, Ishii K, Ikeuchi N, et al. Prospective evaluation of endoscopic ultrasonography-guided double-balloon-occluded gastrojejunostomy bypass (EPASS) for malignant gastric outlet obstruction. Gut 2016;65(2):193–5.
35. Tyberg A, Perez-Miranda M, Sanchez-Ocana R, et al. Endoscopic ultrasound-guided gastrojejunostomy with a lumen-apposing metal stent: a multicenter, inter-national experience. Endosc Int Open 2016;4(3):E276–81.

Lumen-Apposing Metal Stents: Which One and Why?

Matthew W. Stier, MD[a], Irving Waxman, MD[b],*

KEYWORDS

- Lumen-apposing metal stents • Pancreatic fluid collections
- Endoscopic ultrasonography • Transluminal stenting • EUS-guided biliary access
- EUS-guided gallbladder access

KEY POINTS

- Lumen-apposing metal stents (LAMS) have emerged as a primary endoscopic tool for management of complicated pancreatic fluid collections (PFCs) as well as rescue therapy for difficult biliary and gallbladder access.
- Multiple fully covered LAMS have been developed worldwide with a variety of sizes and features for transluminal procedures.
- LAMS delivery includes traditional multistep access via 19-G needle and guidewire insertion as well as a single-step or modified "hot" approach using electrocautery.
- Novel applications for LAMS continue to develop, and next-generation LAMS will be required to optimize their role for endoscopic ultrasound–guided transluminal procedures.

INTRODUCTION

Transluminal endoscopic therapies have evolved rapidly in recent years accompanied by the development of novel endoscopic ultrasound (EUS)-guided stenting devices. In 2012, the Atlanta criteria for acute pancreatitis and the management of pancreatic fluid collections (PFCs) updated terminology and management recommendations, including the importance of transluminal endoscopic approaches in the management of acute pancreatitis and its subsequent complications.[1] Updates to these criteria coincided with the evolution of natural orifice transluminal endoscopic surgery, which was shown to reduce the proinflammatory response and improve composite clinical outcomes in the management of walled off pancreatic necrosis (WON) when

Disclosure Statement: The authors have no financial conflicts of interest to disclose pertaining to this article.
[a] Center for Endoscopic Research and Therapeutics (CERT), The University of Chicago Medicine, 5841 South Maryland Avenue, MC4076, Room M421, Chicago, IL 60637, USA; [b] Center for Endoscopic Research and Therapeutics (CERT), The University of Chicago Medicine, 5700 South Maryland Avenue, MC 8043, Chicago, IL 60637, USA
* Corresponding author.
E-mail address: iwaxman@medicine.bsd.uchicago.edu

compared with surgical necrosectomy.[2–4] Subsequent randomized studies have confirmed endoscopic drainage for pancreatic pseudocysts to reduce hospital length of stay and cost compared with surgical drainage without sacrificing efficacy.[5] Recognition of the potential for nonsurgical approaches to PFCs spurred the development of various stent options for transluminal endoscopic drainage beyond traditional double pigtail plastic stents or metal biliary and esophageal stents used previously.[6,7]

Lumen-apposing metal stents (LAMS) represent a significant advancement in biomedical engineering because of their biflanged design and ability to hold 2 luminal structures in apposition. Their dumbbell shape and wide internal diameter offer theoretic advantages of improved drainage, reduced stent occlusion from necrotic debris, prevention of stent migration, as well as the option for direct endoscopic necrosectomy using a standard forward viewing endoscope when indicated. LAMS have been demonstrated safe (adverse event rates 5%–20%) and effective (clinical success 77%–95%) in expert centers, and their placement under EUS guidance for the management of PFCs is well documented.[8–16]

Despite this technical achievement, there remains a relative paucity of prospective, randomized data proving them superior to older methods. In one review comparing plastic stents with metal stents, including both fully covered self-expanding metal stents (FcSEMS) and LAMS, each stent type performed similarly well in the drainage of pancreatic pseudocysts (85 vs 83%) and WON (70 vs 78%).[17] Bang and colleagues[18] also performed a retrospective study of plastic stents versus LAMS for PFCs and found similar excellent efficacy between stent types (>90%) but a lower cost with plastic stents for pseudocysts.

More recently, multiple retrospective studies have demonstrated a benefit to using LAMS in complicated fluid collections, and the field appears to be progressing toward their use over plastic in this setting.[19] Siddiqui and colleagues[20] retrospectively compared plastic stents to FcSEMS and LAMS for use in WON in 2017, showing that the rate of complete resolution was superior with FcSEMS and LAMS compared with double pigtail stents (90%–95% vs 81%, $P = .001$). The LAMS group in this analysis also required fewer total procedures in comparison with other stent types, potentially offsetting some of the additional up-front cost of the new technology. Other cohort studies have indicated that LAMS use may decrease the need for repeat procedures, total adverse events, salvage surgery, and length of hospital stay when compared with plastic stents for use in complicated fluid collections and WON.[20–23] In light of this information, LAMS are thought to be more efficacious in achieving resolution of WON and are likely cost-effective when used in this setting.[20,21,23–25] Prospective and randomized data are needed to definitively guide their use in the future; however, the obvious design advantages and demonstrated efficacy of LAMS position them to remain the primary means for endoscopic management of complicated PFCs.

TECHNIQUE

Multiple LAMS have been developed and marketed for transluminal applications. First-generation LAMS require a multistep insertion approach without the use of electrocautery. Lesions are accessed via 19-G needle puncture under Doppler ultrasound guidance to ensure avoidance of large vascular structures (**Fig. 1**A). Aspiration of fluid can then be performed as needed for additional diagnostic testing. Needle puncture is followed by placement of a 0.025- or 0.035-inch guidewire to hold the position and subsequent dilation of the tract to facilitate easy passage of the LAMS delivery device (**Fig. 1**B). Dilation can be achieved with needle knife electrocautery or Cystotome

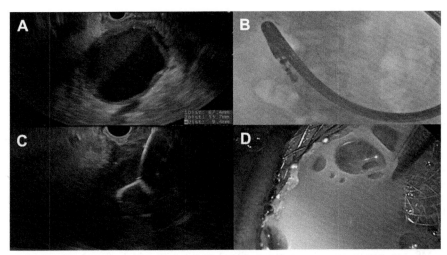

Fig. 1. (*A*) Identification of thick-walled PFC by EUS. (*B*) Insertion of a guidewire into the PFC under fluoroscopy to hold position after 19-G needle stick. (*C*) Distal flange of LAMS deployed under EUS guidance. (*D*) Proximal flange deployment in the bowel lumen with direct endoscopic visualization.

(Cook Medical, Bloomington, IN, not available in the United States) when the fluid collection is clearly compressing the gastrointestinal lumen, Axios delivery device (Boston Scientific, Natick, MA), and/or pneumatic balloon dilation as appropriate. After dilation is performed, the LAMS introducer is passed through the scope, and the distal flange can be deployed transluminally with EUS guidance over the guidewire (**Fig. 1**C). Once the distal flange is fully deployed, gentle tension is applied to oppose the 2 structures before release of the proximal flange under direct endoscopic visualization (**Fig. 1**D). At this point, the stent can be dilated up to its maximal inner diameter as desired by the endoscopist, or left to expand on its own. Some operators also choose to leave a double pigtail stent through the LAMS in hopes of preventing the stent from becoming buried in the cavity wall, migrating, or causing other untoward events.[26]

Second-generation LAMS now include the added option of single-step or modified single-step "hot" insertion using electrocautery. "Hot" insertion is achieved through the application of high-frequency cutting current via diathermic wires that converge on the tip of the device, allowing for transmural access without prior tract dilation.[27] Single-step insertion minimizes over-the-wire exchanges and additional through-the-scope devices and may reduce procedural time while maintaining cost neutrality.[27,28] Electrocautery-assisted LAMS placement has demonstrated similar efficacy when compared with traditional multistep approaches and has been used in PFCs as well as EUS-guided gallbladder drainage and gastrojejunostomy.[12,29–31]

Many operators prefer a hybrid or modified single-step approach that includes puncture of the target with a 19-G needle and guidewire placement before advancement of the LAMS introducer with electrocautery. This technique permits aspiration of fluid for diagnostic testing and confirms appropriate location before LAMS insertion over the guidewire, potentially reducing rates of stent maldeployment. It further avoids tract dilation and excessive over-the-wire exchanges that can add to procedural time and complexity. The modified single-step approach is the preferred LAMS insertion method in most cases, but it remains to be proven if one technique is objectively superior to another for various indications.

AVAILABLE LUMEN-APPOSING METAL STENTS

All LAMS presently on the market are intended for use in PFC management, including pseudocysts and WON. They were designed to improve upon the limitations of double pigtail plastic stents and FcSEMS. Double pigtail stents create a loop in the bowel lumen as well as the adjacent cyst cavity, helping to prevent stent migration. However, their longer length and narrow diameter make them more prone to stent occlusion and increases the need for reintervention, particularly in complicated fluid collections with solid debris.[20,21] Tubular esophageal or biliary stents provide wider diameters, which are thought to offer improved drainage and reduced likelihood of stent occlusion and infection. Tubular stents are prone to stent migration, however, and many recommend their removal after a shorter period.[32] FcSEMS not designed for transluminal procedures also do not anchor tissue planes in apposition, and separation could cause peritonitis because of spillage of luminal contents. Their excessive length further has the potential to impart tissue trauma and can cause delayed bleeding or perforate shallow cavities.[27]

LAMS combine the increased lumen diameter of FcSEMS with wide flanges to prevent stent migration and promote tissue apposition between structures. All available LAMS are composed of a braided nitinol mesh with widely flared or dumbbell-shaped flanges flanking a narrower inner lumen. All models are also fully covered by a silicone membrane. Covered stents help to prevent leakage of air and intestinal contents that can result when partially covered stent migration occurs. The silicone lining also impedes tissue ingrowth, making LAMS easily removable when desired.

Despite their similarities, there are distinct differences between LAMS products in their size, shape, and availability worldwide. The devices offer a variety of delivery mechanisms and features that should be considered when selecting a product for use. Each model is outlined in later discussion and summarized in **Table 1**.

Axios (Boston Scientific)

Perhaps the most widely studied LAMS on the market, and the only stent available in the United States, the Axios stent was developed by Xlumena Inc (Mountain View, CA) and purchased by Boston Scientific (Marlborough, MA) in 2015. It features both single-step "hot" and multistep delivery options, and its introducer features a Luer-lock device that attaches to standard echoendoscopes similar to a fine-needle aspiration device. The delivery system can be controlled by a single operator and is split into a lower catheter control and upper stent control segments. The catheter release mechanism also offers a hard stop between deployment of the distal and proximal flange that is designed to prevent maldeployment of the stent into the cyst lumen.

The Axios stent has a dumbbell or saddle shape with bilateral anchor flanges and comes packaged in a 10.8-Fr delivery device. It is available with inner diameters of 10 mm and 15 mm and a saddle length between flanges of 10 mm. The outer flanges designed to minimize tissue trauma are 21 or 24 mm, respectively (http://www.bostonscientific.com/content/dam/bostonscientific/endo/portfolio-group/AXIOS/axios-cartchart.pdf). The Axios stent has been demonstrated to be feasible for PFC drainage as well as EUS-guided biliary drainage, gallbladder drainage, gastrojejunostomy, and transgastric ERCP (endoscopic retrograde cholangiopancreatography).[11,31,33–37] Removal can be achieved via snare placement around the center lumen with gentle traction through the scope.

Spaxus (Taewoong Medical, Not Available in the United States)

The Niti-S Spaxus is one LAMS model offered by Taewoong Medical (Gimpo-si, South Korea). Its biflange design offers similar atraumatic tissue apposition to that of the Axios

Table 1
Summary of lumen-apposing metal stent products

Stent	Brand	Internal Diameter (mm)	Flange Diameter (mm)	Stent Body Length (mm)	Introducer Diameter (Fr)	Material	Deployment Mechanism	Single Step Delivery?	Studied for
Axios	Boston Scientific	10, 15	21, 24	10	10.8	Nitinol with silicone	TTS, hard stop feature with Luer-lock mechanism	Y	PFC, EUS-BD, EUS-GBD, EUS-GJ
Spaxus	Taewoong	8, 10, 16	23, 25, 31	7	10	Nitinol with silicone	TTS	N	PFC, EUS-GJ, EUS-GBD
NAGI	Taewoong	10, 12, 14, 16	Variable	10, 20, 30	9 or 10	Nitinol with silicone	TTS	N	PFC, EUS-GBD
Aixstent PPS	Leufen	10, 15	25	30	10	Nitinol with silicone	TTS	N	PFC
Hanarostent Plumber	M.I.Tech	10, 12, 14, 16	22, 24, 26, 28	10, 30	10.5	Nitinol with silicone	TTS	N	PFC

Abbreviations: EUS-BD, EUS biliary duct drainage; EUS-GBD, EUS gallbladder drainage; TTS, through-the-scope.

stent and has been applied to PFCs and EUS-guided gallbladder drainage in both animal and human models.[38] Its use has also been evaluated in an animal model for novel endoscopic gastrojejunostomy placement.[39] The Spaxus (Taewoong Medical, Gimposi, South Korea) comes in sizes of 8-, 10-, and 16-mm inner diameter and accompanying outer flange diameter of 23, 25, and 31 mm, respectively. The stent has a total length of 20 mm with a 7-mm distance between flanges. The device is introduced through-the-scope and is housed in a 10-Fr catheter (http://www.stent.net/products/gastroenterology/niti-s-self-expandable-metal-stent/niti-s-biliary-stent/spaxus-stent-pseudocystgallbladder-drainage-2/). It contains radiopaque markers in the ends and center of the stent for visualization under fluoroscopy. Removal is achieved via snare placement with gentle traction.

NAGI (Taewoong Medical, Not Available in the United States)

The second LAMS model offered by Taewoong is the Niti-S NAGI. The NAGI (Taewoong Medical, Gimpo-si, South Korea) is a braided stent with flared ends to maintain tissue apposition and offers a wide variety of sizes available for use. It can be ordered with an inner diameter of 10, 12, 14, or 16 mm as well as lengths of 10, 20, and 30 mm after full expansion. The delivery device is 9 Fr for the 2 smaller sizes and 10 Fr for the 2 larger sizes. It contains radiopaque markers in the ends and center of the stent for visualization under fluoroscopy. The stent also contains a retrieval string designed for easy repositioning and removal (http://www.stent.net/products/gastroenterology/niti-s-self-expandable-metal-stent/niti-s-biliary-stent/nagi-stent-pseudocyst-drainage-2/). The NAGI has been successfully studied for PFC and gallbladder drainage.[15,40–43]

Aixstent (Leufen Medical, Not Available in the United States)

Available in Europe, the Aixstent PPS by Leufen Medical (Berlin, Germany) is a widely flared LAMS that has been studied for drainage of PFCs.[44,45] Its atraumatic folded wire design is intended to minimize tissue trauma at the ends of the stent. It is available in 10- and 15-mm inner diameter with a length of 30 mm from end to end. The bilateral flared ends are 25 mm wide, and it is delivered via a 10-Fr through-the-scope system with radiopaque markers at both ends (https://www.leufen-medical.de/en/aixstentr-gastroenterology/pps-pancreas-pseudocyst-stent.html).

Hanarostent (M.I. Tech, Not Available in the United States)

Hanarostent Plumber by M.I. Tech (Biliary Flange Lasso, Pyeongtaek-si, South Korea) is available in 10-, 12-, 14- or 16-mm inner diameter with usable lengths of 10 or 30 mm. The outer flange diameter ranges from 22 to 28 mm and it is delivered via a 10.5-Fr through-the-scope introducer for PFC drainage.[21] It contains radiopaque markers in the ends and center of the stent for visualization under fluoroscopy (http://www.mitech.co.kr/pds/brochure/Biliary_Flap_Lasso_Pseudocyst.pdf).

STENT SELECTION

PFCs represent a heterogeneous group of disorders, and the decision to use an LAMS as opposed to plastic stents remains a case-by-case choice. Plastic stents appear to have equivalent efficacy for simple pseudocyst drainage and likely are less expensive when used in this setting.[17,18] Complicated cystic fluid collections and WON appear better suited for LAMS use, and superior clinical outcomes have pushed the field in that direction over recent years.[19]

When choosing between available LAMS, there are few data to guide decision making. One study evaluated retrospective outcomes of 43 successive LAMS cases at a single center, finding that no individual LAMS was superior to another in regard to technical success, clinical outcomes, or adverse events. This trial included 10-mm and 15-mm Axios, 12-mm Hanarostent, and 16-mm Niti-S Spaxus at the discretion of the endoscopist, and the use of concomitant nasocystic drainage was not standardized.[21] Another retrospective abstract from 2017 reported outcomes comparing use of second-generation ("hot" Axios) and first-generation (NAGI) LAMS placement at a single center over a 4-year period from 2012 to 2016. They concluded that second-generation LAMS using electrocautery resulted in improved technical success, shorter procedure time, fewer necrosectomies, and shorter length of stay without an increase in cost.[28] It is unknown if this study was standardized for interoperator variability or if the cases occurred at different points in the procedural learning curve. In addition, one study of the NAGI stent showed a lower rate of PFC resolution (76.6%) than that reported in similar LAMS trials. The lower rate of PFC resolution was coupled with a high rate of stent migration (21%), although these variations were not seen in other trials evaluating NAGI stents.[15,16,23,43] There are no currently available prospective or randomized trials comparing size or type of LAMS in regard to technical success, clinical outcomes, or adverse events, and given the range of retrospective data that exists, it is difficult to make data-driven recommendations at this time.

From a practical standpoint, most LAMS are not sold internationally, and local availability or expertise often dictates usage patterns. At this time, only Axios (Boston Scientific) stents are commercially available and approved for use in PFCs in the United States. If single-step or modified single-step approach is preferred, it is important to select an electrocautery-enabled device. Shortened procedural time and lower costs are theoretic advantages of single-step delivery that remain to be proven in prospective trials, and the added utility for experienced operators remains unclear.

In contrast to LAMS type, stent size is often easily modifiable by the endoscopist. Inner diameter and stent length are often variable within each LAMS model. Proximity of the PFC to the intestinal lumen must be considered to ensure apposition can be achieved at a chosen stent or saddle length. The potential need for direct endoscopic necrosectomy should also be considered, because stents larger than 10 to 12 mm would be preferred for optimal passage and maneuverability of a therapeutic forward or side-viewing endoscope. No trials evaluating optimal LAMS diameter or length in relation to clinical outcomes or adverse events have been identified to date.

FUTURE INNOVATIONS

Although the use of LAMS continues to expand, future directions in stent design will be driven by clinical demand and innovative procedural applications. Novel hepatobiliary applications that have been demonstrated feasible include EUS-guided biliary drainage as a rescue therapy for failed ERCP, gallbladder drainage for nonsurgical patients with acute cholecystitis, and EUS-directed transgastric ERCP in the setting of prior gastric bypass.[33,34,36,46–50] There has also been interest in EUS-guided pancreatic duct drainage; however, owing to the large size of current LAMS, this may not be a reasonable strategy without further customization of existing devices.[51] All of these areas require further high-quality research to better define which patients are most likely to benefit from such advanced and risky interventions.

Malignant gastric outlet obstruction is another condition that is well suited for LAMS-directed therapies. EUS-guided endoscopic gastrojejunostomy (EUS-GJ) has the potential to relieve gastric outlet obstruction in patients with advanced cancer who may not be surgical candidates and have failed enteral stenting. There have been multiple studies demonstrating the feasibility of this approach using Axios (Boston Scientific) and Spaxus (Taewoong Medical) stents in animal and human subjects.[31,35,39] Endoscopic gastroenterostomy remains an exciting area of development and may even play a future role in bariatric endoscopy. The ability to easily identify and stabilize the target segment of bowel remains an area of concern and ongoing research.[16,31,52] EUS-GJ may benefit from larger-diameter LAMS that could better allow solid food particles to pass; however, care would need to be taken to avoid dumping syndrome in this setting.

Other intra-abdominal organs could theoretically be accessed endoscopically via LAMS from the stomach or small intestinal lumen for minimally invasive abdominal procedures. At present, this idea is limited by the proximity of distant organs to the intestinal lumen, because current LAMS have an inner length of approximately 10 mm. In order to create stable apposition, devices are needed to better affix these structures to the gastrointestinal lining. Tacking devices would enable this connection and prevent stent migration and loss of apposition, which could cause significant adverse events because of spillage of gastrointestinal contents. Further work is needed in this area before more distant interventions can be considered.

SUMMARY

LAMS represent a major technical advancement in transluminal therapeutic endoscopy. By providing a stable conduit from which a standard endoscope can be easily passed into adjacent structures, novel minimally invasive access and drainage procedures are now possible endoscopically. LAMS have demonstrated a superior efficacy with an acceptable safety profile for use in complicated PFCs and WON when compared with traditional plastic stents and FcSEMS. At present, no high-quality data exist to drive the decision between various LAMS on the market, and these choices are often made based on local availability and expertise. Single-step and modified single-step delivery using electrocautery is available; however, the clinical benefit of "free hand" insertion for current indications is less clear. Proximity to the gastrointestinal lumen and the need for direct endoscopic necrosectomy should be considered when selecting an appropriately sized stent for a given case. LAMS therapeutic potential continues to develop, and future generations of stenting devices will need to be modified to accommodate evolving clinical applications.

REFERENCES

1. Banks PA, Bollen TL, Dervenis C, et al. Classification of acute pancreatitis–2012: revision of the Atlanta classification and definitions by international consensus. Gut 2013;62(1):102–11.
2. Bakker OJ, van Santvoort HC, van Brunschot S, et al. Endoscopic transgastric vs surgical necrosectomy for infected necrotizing pancreatitis: a randomized trial. JAMA 2012;307(10):1053–61.
3. van Santvoort HC, Besselink MG, Bakker OJ, et al. A step-up approach or open necrosectomy for necrotizing pancreatitis. N Engl J Med 2010;362(16):1491–502.
4. Raraty MG, Halloran CM, Dodd S, et al. Minimal access retroperitoneal pancreatic necrosectomy: improvement in morbidity and mortality with a less invasive approach. Ann Surg 2010;251(5):787–93.
5. Varadarajulu S, Bang JY, Sutton BS, et al. Equal efficacy of endoscopic and surgical cystogastrostomy for pancreatic pseudocyst drainage in a randomized trial. Gastroenterology 2013;145(3):583–90.e1.
6. Baron TH, Harewood GC, Morgan DE, et al. Outcome differences after endoscopic drainage of pancreatic necrosis, acute pancreatic pseudocysts, and chronic pancreatic pseudocysts. Gastrointest Endosc 2002;56(1):7–17.

7. Talreja JP, Shami VM, Ku J, et al. Transenteric drainage of pancreatic-fluid collections with fully covered self-expanding metallic stents (with video). Gastrointest Endosc 2008;68(6):1199–203.
8. Sharaiha RZ, Tyberg A, Khashab MA, et al. Endoscopic therapy with lumen-apposing metal stents is safe and effective for patients with pancreatic walled-off necrosis. Clin Gastroenterol Hepatol 2016;14(12):1797–803.
9. Shah RJ, Shah JN, Waxman I, et al. Safety and efficacy of endoscopic ultrasound-guided drainage of pancreatic fluid collections with lumen-apposing covered self-expanding metal stents. Clin Gastroenterol Hepatol 2015;13(4):747–52.
10. Gornals JB, De la Serna-Higuera C, Sánchez-Yague A, et al. Endosonography-guided drainage of pancreatic fluid collections with a novel lumen-apposing stent. Surg Endosc 2013;27(4):1428–34.
11. Siddiqui AA, Adler DG, Nieto J, et al. EUS-guided drainage of peripancreatic fluid collections and necrosis by using a novel lumen-apposing stent: a large retrospective, multicenter U.S. experience (with videos). Gastrointest Endosc 2016;83(4):699–707.
12. Rinninella E, Kunda R, Dollhopf M, et al. EUS-guided drainage of pancreatic fluid collections using a novel lumen-apposing metal stent on an electrocautery-enhanced delivery system: a large retrospective study (with video). Gastrointest Endosc 2015;82(6):1039–46.
13. Vazquez-Sequeiros E, Baron TH, Pérez-Miranda M, et al. Evaluation of the short- and long-term effectiveness and safety of fully covered self-expandable metal stents for drainage of pancreatic fluid collections: results of a Spanish nationwide registry. Gastrointest Endosc 2016;84(3):450–7.e2.
14. Varadarajulu S, Christein JD, Tamhane A, et al. Prospective randomized trial comparing EUS and EGD for transmural drainage of pancreatic pseudocysts (with videos). Gastrointest Endosc 2008;68(6):1102–11.
15. Chandran S, Efthymiou M, Kaffes A, et al. Management of pancreatic collections with a novel endoscopically placed fully covered self-expandable metal stent: a national experience (with videos). Gastrointest Endosc 2015;81(1):127–35.
16. Bank JS, Adler DG. Lumen apposing metal stents: a review of current uses and outcomes. Gastrointest Interv 2017;6:9–14. Available at: http://www.gi-intervention.org/journal/view.html?uid=128&vmd=Full. Accessed January 5, 2018.
17. Bang JY, Hawes R, Bartolucci A, et al. Efficacy of metal and plastic stents for transmural drainage of pancreatic fluid collections: a systematic review. Dig Endosc 2015;27(4):486–98.
18. Bang JY, Hasan MK, Navaneethan U, et al. Lumen-apposing metal stents for drainage of pancreatic fluid collections: when and for whom? Dig Endosc 2017;29(1):83–90.
19. Tyberg A, Kahaleh M. Endoscopic drainage of pancreatic fluid collections: the inevitable shift to metal. Gastrointest Endosc 2016;84(3):458–9.
20. Siddiqui AA, Kowalski TE, Loren DE, et al. Fully covered self-expanding metal stents versus lumen-apposing fully covered self-expanding metal stent versus plastic stents for endoscopic drainage of pancreatic walled-off necrosis: clinical outcomes and success. Gastrointest Endosc 2017;85(4):758–65.
21. Mukai S, Itoi T, Baron TH, et al. Endoscopic ultrasound-guided placement of plastic vs. biflanged metal stents for therapy of walled-off necrosis: a retrospective single-center series. Endoscopy 2015;47(1):47–55.
22. Ang TL, Kongkam P, Kwek AB, et al. A two-center comparative study of plastic and lumen-apposing large diameter self-expandable metallic stents in endoscopic

ultrasound-guided drainage of pancreatic fluid collections. Endosc Ultrasound 2016;5(5):320–7.

23. Bapaye A, Dubale NA, Sheth KA, et al. Endoscopic ultrasonography-guided transmural drainage of walled-off pancreatic necrosis: comparison between a specially designed fully covered bi-flanged metal stent and multiple plastic stents. Dig Endosc 2017;29(1):104–10.

24. Nabi Z, Basha J, Reddy DN. Endoscopic management of pancreatic fluid collections-revisited. World J Gastroenterol 2017;23(15):2660–72.

25. Alali A, Mosko J, May G, et al. Endoscopic ultrasound-guided management of pancreatic fluid collections: update and review of the literature. Clin Endosc 2017;50(2):117–25.

26. Irani S, Kozarek RA. The buried lumen-apposing metal stent: is this a stent problem, location problem, or both? VideoGIE 2016;1(1):25–6.

27. Weilert F, Binmoeller KF. Specially designed stents for transluminal drainage. Gastrointest Interv 2015;4:40–5.

28. Bekkali N, Nayur MK, Leeds JS, et al. Tu 1297 a novel second generation lumen apposing metal stent (LAMS-2) has shorter procedure time, requires fewer necrosectomies and is cost neutral compared to a first generation LAMS for drainage of pancreatic walled off necrosis (WON). Gastrointest Endosc 2017; 85(5S):AB607.

29. Teoh AY, Binmoeller KF, Lau JY. Single-step EUS-guided puncture and delivery of a lumen-apposing stent for gallbladder drainage using a novel cautery-tipped stent delivery system. Gastrointest Endosc 2014;80(6):1171.

30. Patil R, Ona MA, Papafragkakis C, et al. Endoscopic ultrasound-guided placement of AXIOS stent for drainage of pancreatic fluid collections. Ann Gastroenterol 2016;29(2):168–73.

31. Itoi T, Ishii K, Ikeuchi N, et al. Prospective evaluation of endoscopic ultrasonography-guided double-balloon-occluded gastrojejunostomy bypass (EPASS) for malignant gastric outlet obstruction. Gut 2016;65(2):193–5.

32. Binmoeller KF. EUS-guided drainage of pancreatic fluid collections using fully covered self-expandable metal stents. Gastroenterol Hepatol (N Y) 2013;9(7): 442–4.

33. Kedia P, Tyberg A, Kumta NA, et al. EUS-directed transgastric ERCP for Roux-en-Y gastric bypass anatomy: a minimally invasive approach. Gastrointest Endosc 2015;82(3):560–5.

34. Tyberg A, Karia K, Zerbo S, et al. Endoscopic ultrasound-guided choledochojejunostomy with a lumen-apposing metal stent: a shortcut for biliary drainage. Endoscopy 2015;47(Suppl 1 UCTN):E342–3.

35. Tyberg A, Perez-Miranda M, Sanchez-Ocaña R, et al. Endoscopic ultrasound-guided gastrojejunostomy with a lumen-apposing metal stent: a multicenter, international experience. Endosc Int Open 2016;4(3):E276–81.

36. Walter D, Teoh AY, Itoi T, et al. EUS-guided gall bladder drainage with a lumen-apposing metal stent: a prospective long-term evaluation. Gut 2016;65(1):6–8.

37. Walter D, Will U, Sanchez-Yague A, et al. A novel lumen-apposing metal stent for endoscopic ultrasound-guided drainage of pancreatic fluid collections: a prospective cohort study. Endoscopy 2015;47(1):63–7.

38. Moon JH, Choi HJ, Kim DC, et al. A newly designed fully covered metal stent for lumen apposition in EUS-guided drainage and access: a feasibility study (with videos). Gastrointest Endosc 2014;79(6):990–5.

39. Itoi T, Ishii K, Tanaka R, et al. Current status and perspective of endoscopic ultrasonography-guided gastrojejunostomy: endoscopic ultrasonography-guided

double-balloon-occluded gastrojejunostomy (with videos). J Hepatobiliary Pancreat Sci 2015;22(1):3–11.

40. Itoi T, Nageshwar Reddy D, Yasuda I. New fully-covered self-expandable metal stent for endoscopic ultrasonography-guided intervention in infectious walled-off pancreatic necrosis (with video). J Hepatobiliary Pancreat Sci 2013;20(3): 403–6.

41. Yamamoto N, Isayama H, Kawakami H, et al. Preliminary report on a new, fully covered, metal stent designed for the treatment of pancreatic fluid collections. Gastrointest Endosc 2013;77(5):809–14.

42. Rai P, Singh A, Rao RN, et al. First report of endoscopic ultrasound-guided cholecystogastrostomy with a Nagi covered metal stent for palliation of jaundice in extrahepatic biliary obstruction. Endoscopy 2014;46(Suppl 1 UCTN):E334–5.

43. Bapaye A, Itoi T, Kongkam P, et al. New fully covered large-bore wide-flare removable metal stent for drainage of pancreatic fluid collections: results of a multicenter study. Dig Endosc 2015;27(4):499–504.

44. Belle S, Collet P, Post S, et al. Temporary cystogastrostomy with self-expanding metallic stents for pancreatic necrosis. Endoscopy 2010;42(6):493–5.

45. Mangiavillano B, Pagano N, Baron TH, et al. Biliary and pancreatic stenting: devices and insertion techniques in therapeutic endoscopic retrograde cholangiopancreatography and endoscopic ultrasonography. World J Gastrointest Endosc 2016;8(3):143–56.

46. Itoi T, Binmoeller KF, Shah J, et al. Clinical evaluation of a novel lumen-apposing metal stent for endosonography-guided pancreatic pseudocyst and gallbladder drainage (with videos). Gastrointest Endosc 2012;75(4):870–6.

47. Dhir V, Artifon EL, Gupta K, et al. Multicenter study on endoscopic ultrasound-guided expandable biliary metal stent placement: choice of access route, direction of stent insertion, and drainage route. Dig Endosc 2014;26(3):430–5.

48. Park DH, Lee TH, Paik WH, et al. Feasibility and safety of a novel dedicated device for one-step EUS-guided biliary drainage: a randomized trial. J Gastroenterol Hepatol 2015;30(10):1461–6.

49. Sharaiha RZ, Kumta NA, Desai AP, et al. Endoscopic ultrasound-guided biliary drainage versus percutaneous transhepatic biliary drainage: predictors of successful outcome in patients who fail endoscopic retrograde cholangiopancreatography. Surg Endosc 2016;30(12):5500–5.

50. Kunda R, Pérez-Miranda M, Will U, et al. EUS-guided choledochoduodenostomy for malignant distal biliary obstruction using a lumen-apposing fully covered metal stent after failed ERCP. Surg Endosc 2016;30(11):5002–8.

51. Oh D, Park DH, Cho MK, et al. Feasibility and safety of a fully covered self-expandable metal stent with antimigration properties for EUS-guided pancreatic duct drainage: early and midterm outcomes (with video). Gastrointest Endosc 2016;83(2):366–73.e2.

52. Lee HS, Chung MJ. Past, present, and future of gastrointestinal stents: new endoscopic ultrasonography-guided metal stents and future developments. Clin Endosc 2016;49(2):131–8.

Avoidance, Recognition, and Management of Complications Associated with Lumen-Apposing Metal Stents

Stuart K. Amateau, MD, PhD, Martin L. Freeman, MD*

KEYWORDS

- Lumen-apposing metal stent • Complications • Maldeployment • Migration
- Bleeding • Perforation

KEY POINTS

- The lumen-apposing metal stent has evolved endoscopic transluminal therapies, although it has potential complications, including maldeployment, bleeding, perforation, and migration.
- Careful planning and technique mitigate the inherent risks of lumen-apposing metal sent deployment.
- Early recognition and management of lumen-apposing metal stent complications are critical to alleviating morbidity and avoiding mortality.

INTRODUCTION

For decades, most endoscopists feared full-thickness mucosal defects and therefore the field, save for a handful of pioneers, had long been limited to disease management within the gastrointestinal tract. The advent of the lumen-apposing metal stent (LAMS), however, has allowed a broad swath of endoscopists the ability to create controlled full-thickness defects with the intent of connecting the gastrointestinal lumen with other walled compartments or adjacent lumen. With this, advanced gastroenterology now includes the capability of limited extraluminal therapies, including more aggressive transluminal management of walled off necrosis, alternative means of biliary and gallbladder drainage, and creation of enteroenterostomies for alternative routes

Disclosure Statement: Both authors are consultants for Boston Scientific, the manufacturer of the Axios Lumen-Apposing Metal Stent. Neither have financial relationships with companies producing competing products.
University of Minnesota Medical Center, Department of Medicine, Division of Gastroenterology and Hepatology, MMC 36 - 420 Delaware Street SE, Minneapolis, MN 55455, USA
* Corresponding author.
E-mail address: freem020@umn.edu

of per os nutrition or reversal of surgical anatomy.[1–9] As with any advanced intervention, there are risks for complications. These complications can be immediately during the deployment phase or delayed because of the subsequent effects of the intervention and/or stent itself. As with any complication, early recognition remains critical to avoid long-term sequelae and overall poor outcomes. Limited observational data exist evaluating the safety of LAMS for each of the indications; however, maldeployment, bleeding, and free perforation are 3 recognized immediate complications, and migration, bleeding, stent occlusion, and fistulas are delayed concerns. Careful planning, technique, and clinical surveillance will assist in avoiding complications; however, the endoscopist should be ready to manage complications, be it by medical, endoscopic, or surgical interventions.

IMMEDIATE COMPLICATIONS DURING DEPLOYMENT
Cardiopulmonary

Clinical instability and even death may occur acutely following tract creation and stent deployment from aspiration of contents, brisk bleeding, and air embolus. Therefore, all procedures involving LAMS deployment, regardless of the indication, should be performed in conjunction with an anesthesiologist to allow for endotracheal intubation and assistance with clinical monitoring and ventilatory support. Drainage of walled off necrosis or pseudocysts, intraluminal management of strictures, and extraluminal enteroenterostomies all include the risk of fluid reflux, which could be catastrophic if aspirated. Moreover, standard of care involves utilization of carbon dioxide rather than room air for insufflation. Carbon dioxide will both decrease the risk of fatal air emboli, reported in a handful of cases[1] from direct insufflation into a compromised vascular structure, and decrease the morbidity of unforeseen free perforation.

Bleeding

Regardless of the indication, there is a risk of bleeding during stent deployment ranging up to 18% across studies.[1] This may involve rupture of small or large vessels during tract creation, tract dilation, or subsequent spontaneous expansion of the stent. Transluminal placement of the LAMS always involves endoscopic ultrasound (EUS) guidance, allowing for identification of intersecting and nearby vascular structures with adjunct utilization of Doppler. Although choosing the ideal location for placement, the endoscopist should think 3-dimensionally, with concerns beyond the immediate intervening distance and structures, rather to also include the neighboring regions. The covered nature of the stent allows some margin of error because this and the radial expansile properties of the stent allow a degree of constant tamponade. With intramucosal bleeding following stent deployment, subsequent dilation of the stent should be tempered because the slow natural expansion may prompt less immediate bleeding (**Fig. 1**). Immediate bleeding may also occur with rupture of vessels perforating within the adjacent cavity, such as with necrotizing pancreatitis. Preprocedural contrasted imaging frequently will demonstrate large perforating vessels, and frequently those within a few centimeters of the ultrasound probe will be seen on Doppler (**Fig. 2**). Tract creation using free-hand electrocautery tract creation must take these vessels into consideration, and depth of electrocautery application should be controlled so as to not disrupt structures beyond clear endosonographic view.

Maldeployment

Proper deployment of LAMS requires at least partial expansion of both the proximal (outward, deployed second) and the distal (inward, deployed first) flares or anchors.

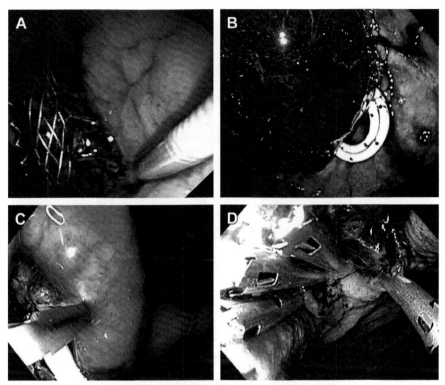

Fig. 1. (*A, B*) Examples of delayed hemorrhage of intraluminal vessel(s) following the creation of cystogastrostomy tracts with (*C, D*) subsequent management endoscopically by LAMS removal and treatment of visible vessel.

Typically, the stent deployment catheter is advanced well within the cavity or adjacent lumen, and the distal anchor is then allowed to expand fully before repositioning the catheter for proximal deployment. This repositioning typically involves tending the distal anchor against the wall of adjacent structure to help ensure the proximal anchor is neither deployed into the adjacent cavity nor within the intervening wall. Frequently, there is decreased space within the proximal cavity (typically the gastrointestinal tract with the echoendoscope) to accommodate optimal positioning, as with a large necrotic cavity extrinsically compressing the natural lumen. This may favor inward deployment, and particular attention should be given to this possibility in such a clinical scenario (**Fig. 3**). Outward migration, on the other hand, occurs most frequently when the intervening distance between targets is greater than 15 mm. Although the cylinder length, or the portion of the stent between the anchors, measures 10 mm across all anchor widths, many have found that tissue compression affords some latitude in terms of distance between targets. The typical sequence in outward migration involves complete distal anchor expansion, with subsequent envelopment of the distal anchor into the tract in the process of attempting to deploy the proximal or outward anchor. In situations whereby stent placement is clinically critical, such as with infected necrosis with clinical instability, however, no appropriate window is found with an intervening distance less than 15 mm, and other stents should be considered, such as traditional double pigtailed plastic stents or full-covered metal biliary stents.

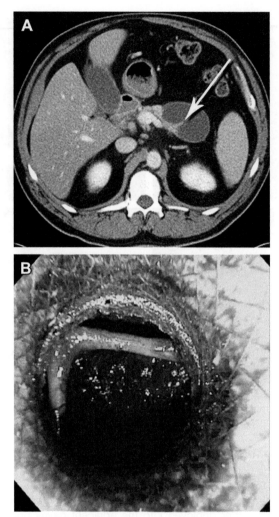

Fig. 2. Demonstration of a large intact vessel (*arrow*) traversing a necrotic cavity initially found on (*A*) preprocedural planning computed tomography and subsequently (*B*) following careful placement of an LAMS.

Free Perforation

Intrinsic to the placement of a lumen metal stent is the creation of a full-thickness mucosal defect, or perforation. The properties of the LAMS seal the perforation so long as the adjacent lumen is contained within a walled structure. In certain circumstances, the walled structure may spontaneously perforate before endoscopic intervention, such as with severe infection of walled off necrosis or acute cholecystitis (**Fig. 4**). Before positioning of the LAMS, a tract must be created, be it by electrocautery or balloon dilation; therefore, subsequent maldeployment of the stents will result in perforation if not addressed in tandem with successful redeployment of an LAMS using the same tract. Such perforations may or may not be clinically significant and occur in upwards of 4% of cases[1]; however, as this cannot be predicted intraprocedurally, efforts should be made to use the original tract. Another consideration should

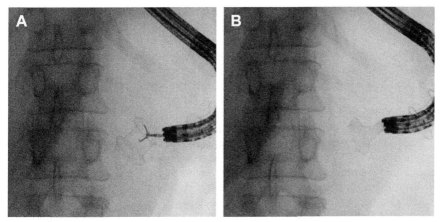

Fig. 3. Inward maldeployment of an LAMS within a necrotic cavity subsequently (*A*) retrieved by passage of a therapeutic gastroscope across a well-positioned LAMS with the stent (*B*) removed through the working channel.

be the apparent adherence of the 2 targets to be linked by the LAMS. Targets that are not fixed to one another present a far greater risk of perforation than those that are, such as with mature necrotic collections intimately apposed to the gastrointestinal tract, or stapled pouches without transection in gastric bypass. Connecting 2 adjacent although nonadherent structures, such as with palliative endoscopic gastrojejunostomy, has increased risk because of the ability of the adjacent structure to move away upon approach, although this has become less of an issue with the advent of one-step electrocautery access.

DELAYED COMPLICATIONS FOLLOWING STENT PLACEMENT OR DURING ENDOSCOPIC THERAPIES
Bleeding

Delayed bleeding in the setting of an LAMS, unlike acute bleeding with deployment, represents a complication that is somewhat beyond the control of the endoscopist.

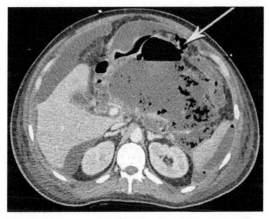

Fig. 4. Demonstration of spontaneous perforation involving a necrotic cavity before any interventional procedure. Arrow points to gas outside of the viscus (perforation).

This is due to the causes, including erosion of the back wall with collapse of necrotic or fluid-filled cavities. Such collapse may not only disrupt small capillaries of the back wall but also lead to injury of larger blood vessel, resulting in pseudoaneurysm and subsequent rupture with profound bleeding.[7] Pseudoaneurysmal bleeding is frequently dramatic and may be first confirmed during contrasted imaging prompted by clinical signs and symptoms of decline and/or during urgent endoscopy (**Fig. 5**). With the former, a blush of contrast may be demonstrated at the site of rupture, whereas during endoscopy, it may be possible to identify the defect in the vascular structure. Bleeding will be brisk, and it is likely that endoscopic visualization would be poor and inadequate for targeted management. Large vessels may also be damaged during transluminal endoscopic therapies, such as during necrosectomy. Large intact perforating vessels may be obscured by solid adjacent necrosis, and therefore, blind passage of stiff penetrating devices, such as forceps, should be avoided. Rather, direct visualization of devices that grasp without penetration, such as snares or suction caps, should be used. It is noted that mild bleeding of the cavity wall during necrosectomy is an acceptable finding, representing clearance of necrotic debris and exposure of viable tissue.

Migration

Frequently LAMS are placed to allow access to the adjacent structure through the stent, as with EUS-directed transgastric endoscopic retrograde cholangiopancrea-tography (ERCP; EDGE) and transluminal endoscopic necrosectomy.[8] Passage of

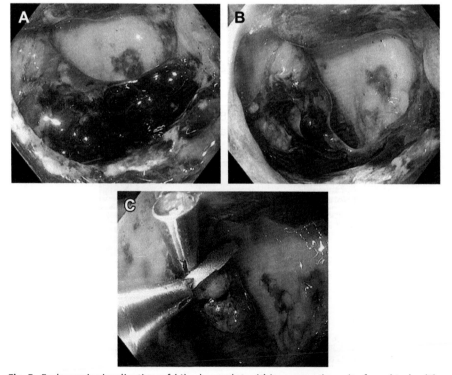

Fig. 5. Endoscopic visualization of (*A*) a large clot within a necrotic cavity found to be (*B*) a bleeding pseudoaneurysm following clot clearance and (*C*) managed serial hemostatic clips.

endoscopes through the stent, in particular, larger-caliber endoscopes, runs a risk for stent dislodgment. If the 2 structures are not adherent, either de novo or over a period of time following stent deployment, such migration may result in free perforation. In this scenario, redeployment of the same or another LAMS using the established tract would be critical. Although it is recommended by the manufacturer to remove the LAMS within 60 days of deployment, this advice is based on theoretic assumptions and pertains to use in necrotizing pancreatitis. On many occasions, these stents may be left in situ far longer, be it due to loss of follow-up or intentional prolonged tract maintenance, and although they tend not to spontaneously migrate, a percentage certainly does. When used for enteroenterostomies or lumen-to-lumen stricture, migration may be either upstream or downstream.[6] Upstream migration typically results in endoscopy with simple stent retrieval, whereas downstream migration may result in benign stasis of the stent near the pylorus or ileocecal valve, or even complete passage per rectum. To the authors' knowledge, migration of the current iterations of LAMS has not resulted in bowel obstruction requiring surgical management.

Endoscopic Transluminal Necrosectomy Specific Complications

Delayed perforation has been found with LAMS during the management of necrotizing pancreatitis.[5] This may be secondary to passage of stiff penetrating devices during necrosectomy, as described earlier for bleeding, or with cavity collapse, prolonged irritation, and subsequent erosion of the back wall by the distal anchor of the metal stent (**Fig. 6**). Without interval computed tomography or MRI, such perforations may be subclinical until discovery during endoscopy. Insufflation across the perforation may result in acute clinical instability and require either endoscopic closure or urgent surgical intervention. Stent occlusion with necrotic contents occurs frequently as the fluid component of the necrotic collection resolves, leaving a heavy burden of semisolid to solid necrotic debris (**Fig. 7**). Although this results in persistent necrosis within the cavity, infected necrosis and sepsis may develop from the ongoing necrotic stasis. For this reason, as well as to mitigate the possibility of back wall injury, management of necrotic cavities should involve radiographic or endoscopic evaluation every 7 to 14 days while the metal stents remain in situ. A percentage of patients with necrotizing pancreatitis has concomitant disconnected pancreatic duct due to complete transection from the necrosis.[1] Endoscopic transluminal drainage (ETD) manages the associated necrotic cavity created by the leak of pancreatic juice from the disconnection;

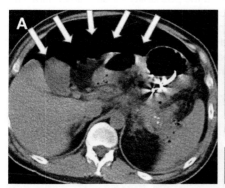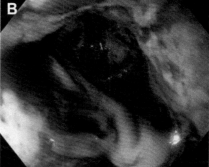

Fig. 6. (*A*) Fluoroscopic (arrows point to gas in the peritoneum) and (*B*) endoscopic demonstration of back wall perforations thought secondary to prolonged irritation by in situ LAMS within collapsed cavities.

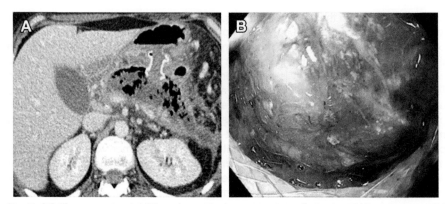

Fig. 7. (A) Fluoroscopic and (B) endoscopic demonstration of stent occlusion due to solid necrosis.

however, with collapse of the cavity and subsequent loss of the pancreaticogastric communication, disconnected duct syndrome may result and the patient may suffer ongoing acute pancreatitis with or without recurrent necrosis. Enterocutaneous fistulas occur in upwards of 5% to 10% of patients with necrotizing pancreatitis managed by LAMS, with the majority in those undergoing both endoscopic and percutaneous drainage techniques.[1] Although these fistulas are not life threatening, they are disruptive and frequently take months and numerous endoscopic procedures to resolve, and on occasion, requiring surgery.

AVOIDANCE OF COMPLICATIONS

As with any endoscopic procedure, careful preprocedural planning and preparation, including review of noninvasive imaging, ensuring appropriate operator expertise, and confirming availability of required equipment, remain the mainstays to decreasing the risks of complication. Contrasted imaging affords the endoscopist the opportunity to plan their window of approach for deployment. Considerations, including distance between adjacent structures, traversing structures such as organs and major vascular structures, and size of targeted cavity, are elucidated and may ultimately lead to pursuit of other methods of intervention (**Fig. 8**). Moreover, compression of the lumen of deployment would be demonstrated hinting at the possibility for difficult proximal anchor expansion. Imaging revealing a significant solid component within a necrotic cavity will alert the operator that the proximal anchor may not completely expand something that may otherwise be confused with poor expansion because of intratract deployment, only the latter of which increases the risk of maldeployment or subsequent migration. Although preprocedural planning is critical, intraprocedural

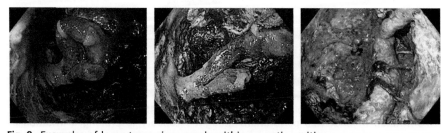

Fig. 8. Examples of large traversing vessels within necrotic cavities.

endosonographic predeployment evaluation is paramount. Insufflation and the endoscope position itself modify the relationships of mobile structures, and in situ views may differ from those anticipated by noninvasive imaging. Choice of window should follow conscientious 3-dimensional endosonographic assessments of adjacent structures and the properties of the target lumen or cavity. If there is any concern about the feasibility of approach, one may consider traditional upfront access by needle and wire passage rather than by catheter-driven electrocautery. This provides the opportunity to abort and avoid perforation with the wider-caliber catheter passage. Moreover, passage of an electrocautery catheter over a guidewire decreases the risk of back wall injury in the scenario of smaller targets, as with gallbladder access, as well as maintains the tract in the event of maldeployment. Specifically, with the wire in place, the maldeployed stent may be captured by forceps and removed through the endoscope and a second stent then positioned across the tract for appropriate deployment. In terms of intraprocedural migration, the current iterations of LAMS available in the United States have a maximal caliber of 15 mm. Immediate passage of endoscopes across an LAMS seated in a fresh tract has the risk of iatrogenic migration in particular with endoscopes with larger outer diameters. Therefore, some have favored the use of nontherapeutic endoscopes for upfront ERCP with EDGE, tandem immediate necrosectomy, or other acute interventions across the LAMS. With ETD stent, occlusion and sepsis may occur as the fluid component resolves and necrotic debris obstructs the lumen of the stent. Moreover, as mentioned earlier, such collapse of the cavity may also result in back wall injury against the inward anchor and disconnected duct syndrome. Shorter-interval radiographic and/or endoscopic evaluation would provide evidence of imminent or ongoing stent occlusion and cavity collapse, prompting stent revision, removal, or clearance. Despite lack of data to date, many favor deployment of soft double pig-tailed stents within the LAMS to theoretically decrease stent occlusion, back wall trauma, and loss of tract with complete cavity collapse. As the iterations of LAMS continue to evolve, for instance, with increasing caliber options, these variables will likely be affected, although it remains unclear if these will have more favorable or unfavorable characteristics.

RECOGNITION AND MANAGEMENT
Bleeding

Regardless of the operator's preparation and expertise, complications will occur. Although these complications to some extent are unavoidable and acceptable, ignoring or misinterpreting signs of complications is inexcusable. Furthermore, early recognition of complications provides the best chance for minimizing or even removing morbidity related to the procedure. Injury to intramucosal vessels during transluminal stent placement will be evident immediately, although not all require intervention because the properties of the stent allow tamponade. Bleeding that is brisk from under the stent, seen across the stent covering, should be observed endoscopically for a short period of time. With continuation, removal of the stent is not recommended at this juncture; rather, the endoscopist may consider directed submucosal injection of 1:10,000 (1mg/10ml) epinephrine. This in combination with stent tamponade should mitigate defects of smaller vascular structures. Brisk bleeding from within the adjacent cavity or lumen through the stent should alert the operator of possible injury to a perforating larger vascular structure, either preexisting and now revealed, or iatrogenic with catheter passage. Again, endoscopic options are relatively limited, although one may consider passage of a forward viewing endoscope across the stent into the cavity for evaluation and possible therapy as one would with delayed bleeding.

If visualization within the cavity is feasible, the bleeding source may be identified and hemostasis attempted with through-the-scope hemostatic clips with or without injection of dilute epinephrine. When bleeding is immediate and endoscopically uncontrolled, or when delayed, computed tomography with intravenous contrast is desirable, assuming renal function allows. This may demonstrate injury to vascular structures, such as pseudoaneurysms with a blush of contrast, and/or suggest current hemostasis. As with any interventional procedure, anticoagulation should be held for 2 to 3 days following the procedure if comorbidities allow, in particular, with suggestion of iatrogenic injury. Hemoglobin should be followed and with evidence of subsequent continued or delayed bleeding, anticoagulation would be contraindicated, and other options, such as lowering the therapeutic window and placement of an inferior vena cava filter, should be considered. With evidence of ongoing bleeding from larger vascular structures not amenable to endoscopic therapy, consultation of experienced interventional radiologists for targeted angiography and vascular coiling would be the next appropriate step, although in rare instances the vascular structure may be evident by endosonography and the coiling may be performed by experienced endoscopists (**Fig. 9**). Occasionally, intraprocedural bleeding will be critical and accompanied by hemodynamic instability and abdominal compartment syndrome. In these instances, urgent intraprocedural consultation with experienced surgeons is indicated for consideration of exploratory laparotomy and hemostatic source control.

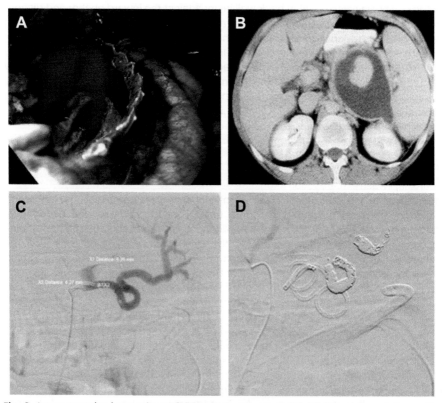

Fig. 9. Large vascular hemorrhage from within a cavity with (*A*) blood found across the LAMS and subsequently demonstrated on (*B*) contrasted CT with a blush of contrast within the cavity and later during (*C*) angiography, prompting (*D*) tandem coiling for hemostasis.

Maldeployment

Proper deployment of LAMS involves at least partial expansion of the body and complete expansion of both anchors with communication to the desired adjacent lumen or cavity. Maldeployment therefore is failure to achieve any of these objectives and may occur, as noted earlier, because of poor availability or selection of deployment window, and should be immediately recognized. With poor expansion of an anchor due to longer than desired tract, one may consider removal of the stent in favor of selection of another more desirable window, assuming one exists. In this scenario, however, the operator may create a free perforation and will need to then consider closing at least the stomach defect and recognize the possibility that this still may result in content spillage into the abdominal cavity if the compartments were not adhered. Another option would be to salvage the tract with deployment of either a second stent in stent LAMS or removal of the LAMS over a wire and subsequent placement of a 10-mm fully covered metal biliary stent (FCMBS), perhaps one with proximal and distal antimigration flanges. Maldeployment may also involve complete misdeployment of the stent within the adjacent lumen or cavity or within the lumen of origin. Again, salvage of the initial tract is preferable because it would avoid the risk of free perforation, and therefore, as recommended previously, needle access for wire passage before stent deployment should be considered in situations whereby factors suggest a difficult placement. This wire may then be used to properly place an LAMS or FCMBS. Following placement, the maldeployed stent may be retrieved, either through the well-positioned LAMS or from the lumen of origin, and if with the former, consideration should be given to removal through the working channel of a therapeutic endoscope so as to avoid dislodging the well-positioned stent.

Perforation

As noted previously, perforation although typically immediate from tract creation may rarely be delayed from back wall trauma secondary to stent erosion. Both instances are recognized by clinical instability, which may be acute and dramatic, and confirmed by imaging. If immediate, fluoroscopy required for placement should be used to evaluate for subdiaphragmatic gas, and if detected, continued insufflation should be limited. If the adjacent compartments are adhered and the tract defect is without a well-positioned LAMS, the operator may consider closure of the proximal defect with an over-the-scope clip, a series of hemostatic clips, or endoscopic suturing, assuming the patient remains hemodynamically stable (**Fig. 10**). Carbon dioxide should resorb within minutes with appropriate closure, and significant quantities of residual gas on fluoroscopy should reflex an intraoperative surgical consultation. Delayed perforation because of back wall erosion from stent irritation in the setting of cavity collapse will typically require surgical laparotomy, however rarely, may be managed by endoscopic closure across the tract with through-the-scope clips assuming patient stability. Endoscopic suturing and over-the-scope clips are not options because of the incompatibility of the width of these devices with the tract caliber. Incompletely mature necrotic collections, in particular, those communicating with the root of the mesentery, should be approached with care because these frequently result in perforation requiring surgical management.

Delayed Stent-Specific Complications

Beyond back wall stent erosion leading to bleeding and/or perforation, LAMS may become obstructed with necrosis when used for necrotizing pancreatitis or migrate in any scenario into the adjacent compartment or into the gastrointestinal tract in continuity. When obstructed with necrosis, further spontaneous drainage will halt, and in

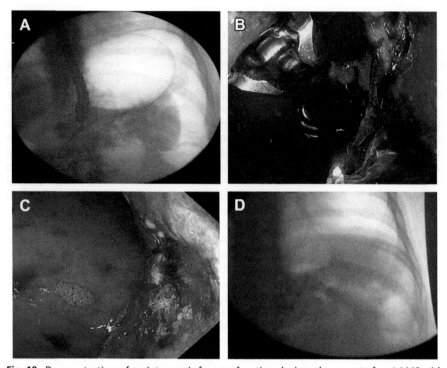

Fig. 10. Demonstration of an iatrogenic free perforation during placement of an LAMS with (*A*) a large amount of gas beneath the left diaphragm. As the cavities were adherent (*B, C*), endoscopic suture closure of the endoscopic defect was performed with (*D*) near immediate resolution of the gas on fluoroscopy.

some scenarios, sepsis will occur. Management involves careful postprocedure planning with scheduled endoscopic transluminal necrosectomy (ETN) within several days of the initial ETD if there is a heavy solid necrotic burden. At times, despite reasonable planning, evidence of early obstruction and sepsis occurs, necessitating urgent ETN. Clearance of necrosis is facilitated by removal of the LAMS as the distal inward anchor catches larger pieces; however, care should be taken early in the process before removal of the LAMS, in particular, if the 2 compartments were not adhered de novo. Migration of the stent into the bowel may require endoscopic or rarely surgical retrieval; however, the authors have found that currently available LAMS tend to linger at natural narrowings, including the pylorus, ileocecal valve, and anus, allowing for endoscopic management. Migration into adjacent cavities presents a slightly more complicated scenario if the cavity has collapsed and the tract has begun to close. Ideally, the tract would be dilated and the stent grasped and removed using both endoscopic and fluoroscopic guidance. Stent migration into persistent adjacent cavity, without a residual tract, necessitates repeat tract creation and stent placement, following which the malpositioned stent may be recovered. There have also been reports of LAMS buried within the tract and mechanical compression of the common duct secondary to cavity collapse and cystoduodenostomy.

Fistulas

Low-output enterocutaneous fistulas represent one of the more common complications of stent deployment in patients with necrotizing pancreatitis, with the majority seen in those having concomitant percutaneous drainage. These fistulas are disruptive and may take months to resolve despite numerous endoscopic and percutaneous procedures. Rarely, they require surgical management. As with any enterocutaneous fistula, diversion of body fluids in combination with management of both the luminal and the cutaneous sites of defect underlie the successful therapy. Suturing or clipping the lumen defect alone typically fails and requires at least tandem slow withdrawal of the percutaneous drain to allow sequential tract closure. Other endoscopic maneuvers, such as placement of a fistula plug in short tracts and deployment of fibrin glue, have been attempted with less than desirable overall outcomes.

SUMMARY

The LAMS has evolved endoscopic transluminal therapies, although it has potential complications, including maldeployment, bleeding, perforation, migration, and several risks specific to necrotizing pancreatitis. Careful planning and technique mitigate these inherent risks of LAMS deployment; however, setbacks occur even in the most experienced of hands. Therefore, early recognition and management of these complications are critical to alleviating morbidity and avoiding mortality. Management frequently requires multidisciplinary effort, including advanced endoscopic technique and consultation of interventional radiologic and surgical colleagues.

REFERENCES

1. van Brunschot S, Fockens P, Bakker OJ, et al. Endoscopic transluminal necrosectomy in necrotizing pancreatitis: a systematic review. Surg Endosc 2014;28(5): 1425–38.
2. Binninella E, Kunda R, Dollhopf M, et al. EUS-guided drainage of pancreatic fluid collections using a novel lumen-apposing metal stent on an electrocautery-enhanced delivery system: a large retrospective study. Gastrointest Endosc 2015;82:1039–46.
3. Shah RJ, Shah JN, Waxman I, et al. Safety and efficacy of endoscopic ultrasound-guided drainage of pancreatic fluid collections with lumen-apposing covered self-expanding metal stents. Clin Gastroenterol Hepatol 2015;13:747–52.
4. Tyberg A, Saumoy M, Sequeiros EV, et al. EUS-guided versus percutaneous gallbladder drainage: isn't it time to convert? J Clin Gastroenterol 2018;52(1): 79–84.
5. Sharaiha RZ, Tyberg A, Khashab MA, et al. Endoscopic therapy with lumen-apposing metal stents is safe and effective for patients with pancreatic walled-off necrosis. Clin Gastroenterol Hepatol 2016;14(12):1797–803.
6. Bazerbachi F, Heffley JD, Abu Dayyeh BK, et al. Safety and efficacy of coaxial lumen-apposing metal stents in the management of refractory gastrointestinal luminal strictures: a multicenter study. Endosc Int Open 2017;5(9):E861–7.
7. Ryan BM, Venkatachalapathy SV, Huggett MT, et al. Safety of lumen-apposing metal stents (LAMS) for pancreatic fluid collection drainage. Gut 2017;66(8):1530–1.
8. Tyberg A, Nieto J, Salgado S, et al. Endoscopic ultrasound (EUS)-directed trans-gastric endoscopic retrograde cholangiopancreatography or EUS: mid-term analysis of an emerging procedure. Clin Endosc 2017;50(2):185–90.
9. Bang JY, Hasan M, Navaneethan U, et al. Lumen apposing metal stents (LAMS) for pancreatic fluid collection (PFC) drainage: may not be business as usual. Gut 2017;66(12):2054–6.

Endoscopic Closure of Gastrointestinal Fistulae and Leaks

Jaehoon Cho, MD[a], Ara B. Sahakian, MD[b],*

KEYWORDS

- Lumen-apposing metal stent • Fistula • Leak

KEY POINTS

- Endoscopic fistula closure offers a minimally invasive alternative to surgery when conservative measures fail.
- Endoscopic therapies for management of fistula and leaks include stenting, clipping, full-thickness suturing, and use of tissue adhesives. These therapies continue to evolve and show promising results.
- The lumen apposing metal stent (LAMS) has provided the endoscopist the ability to create iatrogenic fistulae to treat disease states.
- Fistulae resulting from the LAMS have not been routinely closed after the LAMS removal. Further study is warranted to determine whether residual fistula closure may be necessary in certain instances, such as transgastric fistula in Roux-en-Y gastric bypass.

INTRODUCTION

A gastrointestinal (GI) fistula is an abnormal connection between an abdominal organ and another organ (internal fistula) or the body surface (external fistula). These fistulae may arise from malignant or inflammatory conditions, or may be iatrogenic, occurring after surgery, endoscopic therapy, or radiation therapy. Traditionally, conservative measures and surgical therapy has been the mainstay of treatment of GI fistulae. However, surgical therapy tends to be complex and is plagued by high rates of morbidity.[1] In recent years, advances in interventional endoscopic techniques have altered the management paradigm for GI fistula, allowing for an additional option before considering surgery.

Disclosure Statement: There were no grants or financial contributions to this article. There is no conflict of interest to state from any of the listed authors pertaining to this article.
[a] Department of Internal Medicine, Los Angeles County and University of Southern California Medical Center, 2020 Zonal Avenue, IRD 620, Los Angeles, CA 90033, USA; [b] Division of Gastrointestinal and Liver Diseases, University of Southern California Keck School of Medicine, 1510 San Pablo Street, Los Angeles, CA 90033, USA
* Corresponding author.
E-mail address: Arasahak@med.usc.edu

Gastrointest Endoscopy Clin N Am 28 (2018) 233–249
https://doi.org/10.1016/j.giec.2017.11.010
1052-5157/18/© 2017 Elsevier Inc. All rights reserved.

Development of new endoscopic techniques, such as GI stenting, suturing, clip application, and use of tissue adhesives, have had a significant impact on management of GI fistulae. The advancement of endoscopic technology, including the lumen apposing metal stent (LAMS), has allowed for the deliberate creation of GI fistula to perform endoscopic therapy that previously could not be achieved. These techniques continue to evolve and require further study for optimization of efficacy. The aim of this article is to examine the rapidly evolving area of endoscopic fistula closure and its relation to LAMS.

DIAGNOSIS

The first step in diagnosing a GI defect is through examination and medical history. Common symptoms include pain (initially localized but may become diffuse) and fever[2]; however, some patients may be completely asymptomatic. Once the suspicion for GI fistula or leak exists, the source and route must be established to determine the appropriate intervention.

Enterocutaneous fistula may be diagnosed based on appearance. Enterocutaneous fistulas may present with abnormal drainage from the skin, such as purulence or intestinal contents. Definitive diagnosis requires cross-sectional imaging, such as computed tomography (CT), MRI, or contrast fistulogram, demonstrating an abnormal connection between bowel and another organ.[3] When fistulae are too small for imaging, dye injected via catheter or during endoscopy can aid in diagnosis. Evidence of staining in wound drainage, urine, feces, or from the vagina may confirm the presence of enteric fistula.[4]

Internal GI fistulae are more difficult to diagnose than enterocutaneous fistulae. Comprehensive study of the anatomic defect requires imaging modalities such as contrast fistulogram, CT, MRI, or radionuclide testing. For contrast studies, barium is the medium of choice for its ability to remain undiluted and define mucosal surfaces (**Fig. 1**). However, extravasated barium may induce an inflammatory reaction. Therefore, a water-soluble medium should be considered if there is a concern for GI perforation or leak.[5] In addition, carbon dioxide is recommended for insufflation during

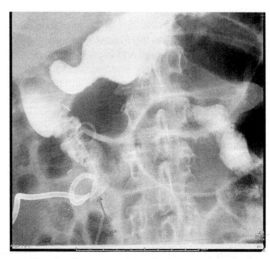

Fig. 1. Contrast upper GI series demonstrating a leak (*arrow*) at the junction of the second and third portions of the duodenum after surgical resection of a sarcoma.

fistulogram because the gas may cross into the peritoneum or mediastinum via the defect.[6] Ultrasound is often used as a primary screening modality; however, it is operator dependent and the may be hindered by the body habitus of the patient. Therefore, CT may be useful in providing more standardized information independent of body habitus and operator skill.[4]

CONSERVATIVE MANAGEMENT

The first step in conservative management of GI disruption includes resuscitation and management of sepsis, if present. Disturbance in the lining of the GI tract can lead to a hypovolemic state secondary to bowel losses, as well as intraabdominal third spacing related to inflammation.[7] Volume resuscitation and correction of electrolytes through intravenous fluid replacement should be initiated. The fluid therapy of choice is isotonic saline supplemented with potassium. In cases of duodenal fistulae, bicarbonate may be added if metabolic acidosis occurs.

Septic complications often represent the primary cause of mortality related to GI fistulae.[8] Successful control of sepsis depends on elimination of septic foci via image-guided drainage and antibiotic therapy.[9] Percutaneous drainage of fluid collections by interventional radiology is considered a mainstay of therapy.[10] Patients with uncontrolled sepsis may benefit from surgical washout of the abdominal cavity or diverting proximal stoma.[11] However, the optimal treatment of the hemodynamically stable patient is to prevent surgery by using conservative measures and minimally invasive therapies.

Malnutrition is another major contributing factor to morbidity and mortality from GI disruption.[12,13] Malnutrition is not only a predictive factor for mortality but also predictive of fistula closure. Signs of malnutrition include body weight loss greater than 10% or presence of hypoproteinemia.[14] Malnutrition is caused by protein-rich GI secretions, increased catabolism secondary to sepsis, and decreased oral-intake. Nutritional support should begin when patient has been stabilized from a fluid and acid-base standpoint. Enteral and/or parenteral feeds are essential in providing nutritional support. Total parenteral nutrition (TPN) has been mainstay of conservative management for GI fistulae. Conservative management with TPN has been shown to decrease fistula output by up to 50% and promote a favorable condition for spontaneous closure.[15] However, TPN is limited by serious complications, such as metabolic disorders and infections. Therefore, the route of nutritional supplementation may depend on whether enteral nutrition is feasible because evidence suggests its superiority over parenteral nutrition in terms of safety and efficacy.[16,17]

Reducing fistula output is considered a critical aspect of conservative management of GI fistulae. Although there is a paucity of data showing a definitive association between controlling fistula output and rate of spontaneous closure, it is associated with maintenance of volume, electrolyte balance, and nutritional status.[7] Pharmacologic agents for reducing fistula output include somatostatin analogues such as octreotide. Octreotide is the only synthetic analogue available in the United States, but its clinical use is limited by a short half-life.[18] Multiple case series have reported decrease in fistula output of up to 70% with pharmacologic agents.[19,20] However, prospective placebo-controlled trials failed to show significant difference in rate of fistula closure and mortality with the use of somatostatin and its analogues.[21–24]

Spontaneous closure of GI fistulae may be seen after 5 to 6 weeks with conservative management without radiological or surgical interventions. Factors contributing to an increased rate of spontaneous closure include low fistula output, length of tract greater than 2 cm, and proximal bowel involvement.[5,25] Anatomic factors that may adversely affect spontaneous closure include lateral fistula, bowel abscess, and distal obstruction of bowel.[4] When conservative measures fail, endoscopic therapy should be considered as an adjunct treatment to aid in fistulae closure.

ENDOSCOPIC STENTS

Endoscopic stents are cylindrical devices used to preserve or reestablish luminal patency.[26] For GI defects, the role of a stent is to seal the fistula and to divert GI contents away from the site of leakage. Compared with conservative treatment, stent placement results in earlier oral intake, a shorter hospital stay and lower in-hospital mortality.[27] There are 3 types of stents used to manage full-thickness GI defect: the self-expandable plastic stent (SEPS), the self-expandable metal stent (SEMS), and the biodegradable stent (BDS).

The BDS is an absorbable stent that degrades in 6 to 24 weeks. Degradation is accelerated by acid exposure. Therefore, acid-suppressive therapy may be warranted in certain situations.[28] The radial force of a BDS is maintained for 6 weeks following deployment before it is degraded. However, the radial force of BDS is weaker than that of SEMS.[29] BDS were first used in 2008, but are currently not available for use in full-thickness GI defect repair in the United States.

The SEPS consists of a polyester body covered with silicone to prevent tissue ingrowth and polyester braids on the surface to prevent stent migration. Radio-opaque markers are positioned at the middle and ends of the stent to allow for visualization of this nonmetallic device during fluoroscopy. The initial purpose of the SEPS was for treatment of esophageal strictures.[30] The SEPS is effective in sealing a defect in the bowel wall; however, it has a propensity for migration.[31] In multiple retrospective series, up to 50% of the SEPS placed were complicated by migration.[32,33] A SEPS placed in upper GI tract rarely passes beyond the pylorus. However, a SEPS placed in lower GI tract may migrate proximally or distally, leading to incidences of perforation and obstruction.[6] In addition to issues with migration, a SEPS requires mounting on a delivery system before deployment, making the process complicated compared with a SEMS, which is ready for use.[34] For these reasons, the use of the SEPS has been largely been replaced by use of the SEMS.

The SEMS can be delivered either through-the-scope (TTS) or over-the-wire (OTW), depending on the type of stent and location of delivery. Currently, colonic stents and duodenal stents are available as uncovered stents, which are delivered through TTS. An esophageal SEMS may be uncovered, partially covered, or fully covered and is generally delivered OTW, although TTS esophageal stents are now commercially available. A SEMS can be made of either elgiloy or nitinol. Elgiloy is an alloy composed of cobalt, nickel, and chromium, providing high radial force and corrosion resistance. Nitinol is an alloy of nickel and titanium, allowing flexibility for placement at sharp angles but with less radial force than a SEMS made of elgiloy (**Fig. 2**).[34,35]

Uncovered SEMS are not indicated in management of GI tract fistulae because they do not have the ability to seal the defect or divert bowel contents. Thus, the lack of availability of a covered enterocolonic SEMS poses a challenge to management of fistulae in these regions. However, off-label use of covered esophageal stents for management of enterocolonic fistulae has shown promising results.[36]

In several retrospective series, the fully covered SEMS (FCSEMS) has been reported to have a migration rate of up to 30%.[37–39] FCSEMS with endoscopic suture fixation has been proposed to further decrease the rate of migration (**Fig. 3**). A meta-analysis by Law and colleagues[40] reviewed 14 studies from 2011 to 2016 to investigate the migration rate of the SEMS after endoscopic suture fixation. Migration occurred in

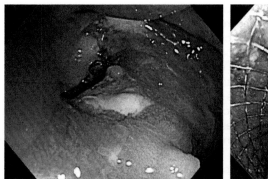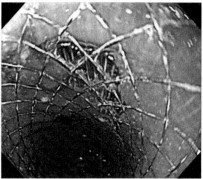

Fig. 2. Treatment of colocutaneous fistula in the sigmoid colon using a fully covered SEMS (FCSEMS). Fistula before stent placement (*left*). Fistula seen through the stent covering (*right*).

15.9% of cases. Endoclip fixation of the FCSEMS has been reported[41]; however, data on the efficacy of this technique are limited.

The partially covered SEMS (PCSEMS) has a membrane covering the body of the stent, but the proximal and distal ends are uncovered, allowing for tissue ingrowth in these regions. Theoretically, the tissue ingrowth decreases the rate of migration. A pooled analysis of 20 retrospective studies by van Halsema and van Hooft[42] looked at the outcomes of stent placement for benign esophageal leaks, perforations, and fistulae. A total of 643 subjects were treated with the SEMS. The overall migration rate was 16.5%. The migration rate for the FCSEMS was 21.8% as opposed to 10.6% for the PCSEMS. Although the migration rate may be lower, PCSEMS may be difficult to remove after the leak or fistula has resolved. Placing a SEPS within a PCSEMS is a technique that has been used to remove them. The theory is that the SEPS leads to pressure necrosis of the ingrown tissue at the margins of the PCSEMS, allowing for removal after a period of several weeks. A retrospective study by Alazmi and colleagues[43] looking at efficacy of the SEPS-assisted retrieval process showed clinical success with leak closure in 76% of the subjects (13 out of 17 subjects). More importantly, all stents were successfully removed with only minor bleeding in 2 (12%) of the 17 subjects. The following year, Swinnen and colleagues[44] demonstrated efficacy of the SEPS-assisted retrieval process in a study consisting of 88 subjects. The rate of successful removal was 97.8%. Resolution of leaks and perforation

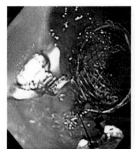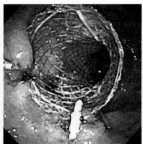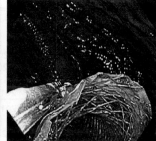

Fig. 3. An FCSEMS with suture fixation for treatment of duodenal leak or fistula. Endoscopic suturing using OverStitch device (*left*). Successful endoscopic fixation of an FCSEMS (*middle*). Removal of FCSEMS with a forceps after proximal migration into the stomach (*right*).

was 77.6%, which was similar to the study conducted by Alazmi and colleagues.[43] In this study, the PCSEMS had migration rate of 11.1% with major complications (bleeding, perforation) in 5.9% of the cases. Most experts recommend PCSEMS removal by the SEPS-assisted retrieval process 6 to 10 weeks after stent placement.

One retrospective study compared the efficacy of the FCSEMS and the PCSEMS in treatment of esophageal leaks, fistulae, and perforations. All stents were removed using a standard single-channel or double-channel therapeutic upper endoscope and rat-tooth forceps. Among the 54 subjects included in the study, 117 stents were placed with technical success in all cases. Primary closure was defined as complete closure of the disruption after index stent removal; whereas secondary closure was defined as the need for repeat stenting. Primary closure was accomplished in 74% of the subjects with 83% clinical success, including secondary closures. The study did not show any advantage of the FCSEMS compared with the PCSEMS.[45] A similar study comparing the fully and partially covered SEMS led to same conclusion: both stent types had similar outcomes for repair of esophageal fistulas and leaks.[46] A retrospective study comparing 3 types of stents (FCSEMS, PCSEMS, and SEPS) for benign esophageal rupture or leak evaluated 52 subjects with 83 stents. The clinical success rate was as follows: PCSEMS 73%, FCSEMS 83%, and SEPS 83%. There was no statistically significant difference in clinical success between the 3 types of stents. Therefore, the investigators concluded that the choice of stent should depend on risks of stent migration and tissue ingrowth.[47] Studies evaluating the efficacy the SEMS for treatment of GI leaks or fistula are summarized in **Table 1**.

CLIPS

Endoscopic clips have multiple roles in repair of GI tract disruptions. Clips can be used to fix stents to the lumen to prevent migration, seal leaks, and close fistulae.[56] Two types

Table 1
Studies investigating the efficacy of stents for fistula and leak repair

Location	Study	Type of Stent (Subset of Subjects)	Number of Subjects	Short-Term Closure of Leaks or Fistulae (%)
Esophagus	Bakken et al,[37] 2010	FCSEMS	56	38
	El Hajj et al,[45] 2014	PCSEMS plus FCSEMS	44	73
	Eloubeidi et al,[38] 2011	FCSEMS	35	31
	Buscaglia et al,[31] 2011	FCSEMS	31	80
	Suzuki et al,[48] 2016	PCSEMS plus FCSEMS	19	74
Stomach	Christophorou et al,[49] 2015	FCSEMS (82) plus PCSEMS (14) plus SEPS (8)	110	74
	El Mourad et al,[50] 2013	PCSEMS	47	87
	Eisendrath et al,[51] 2007	PCSEMS	21	62
	Salinas et al,[52] 2006	PCSEMS	17	94
	Garofalo et al,[53] 2017	FCSEMS	11	91
Duodenum/ Colon	Lamazza et al,[54] 2015	FCSEMS (19) plus UCSEMS (3)	22	86
	DiMaio et al,[55] 2012	FCSEMS (4) plus PCSEMS (1)	5	80

Abbreviations: FCSEMS, fully covered self-expandable metal stent; PCSEMS: partially covered self-expandable metal stent; UCSEMS, uncovered self-expandable metal stent.

of clips have been used for closure of fistulae: the TTS clip (TTSC) and the over-the-scope clip (OTSC). The TTSC is reserved for closing smaller luminal defects, measuring less than 2 cm in size.[6,57] The advantages of the TTSC over the OTSC are ease of use, ability to rotate, and ability to reopen if needed. However, approximation of luminal defects when the surrounding tissue is inflamed or necrotic may be difficult with the TTSC. The TTSC may be limited in closure of fistulae due to the width of the clip arms and the limited pressure that can be applied to the tissue.[58] The TTSC is designed to spontaneously dislodge, which may limit its efficacy for treatment of fistulae.

Use of the OTSC is an attempt to overcome the limitations of the TTSC for closure of GI tract disruptions. It has wider clip arms, allowing for recruitment of more tissue, which is grasped with greater force.[59] Assembly and deployment is similar to that of a variceal band ligation device. The region of interest is suctioned into a cap and the clip is deployed by turning a knob attached to the hub of the endoscope (**Fig. 4**). The entire margin of the defect must be within the cap; grasping the forceps that are inserted through the working channel can assist with this. The OTSC has been reported to repair gastric defects up to 20 mm in diameter. In the colon, an OTSC has been shown to repair lesions up to 30 mm in diameter in an ex vivo experiment. Larger defects may require more than 1 OTSC or an additional TTSC to achieve adequate closure.[60]

Clinical outcomes for OTSC closure of GI fistulae and leaks have been studied in multiple retrospective studies with a success rate of 75% to 89% for closure of fistulae and leaks.[61,62] However, long-term follow-up is limited. One study by Law and colleagues[63] evaluated 47 cases of chronic GI fistulae repaired with an OTSC. Initial technical success was achieved in 89% of the cases, which is similar to outcomes seen in other case series. However, in these cases of initial technical success, 46% of the subjects developed a recurrent fistula in the same location in a median of 39 days. These data call into question the long-term clinical efficacy of the OTSC for management of fistulae. Studies demonstrating efficacy of the OTSC for closure of leaks or fistulae are summarized in **Table 2**.

There are several limitations to use of endoscopic clips for closure of fistulae. A TTSC may not properly grasp the tissue surrounding the fistula if it is inflamed or edematous. A TTSC can also prematurely and spontaneously dislodge, limiting its duration of action. Conversely, OTSC removal can be challenging in cases of clinical failure, when a secondary intervention may be warranted. Several methods of OTSC removal have been reported, including use of argon plasma coagulation or a bipolar cutting device to fracture the clip, or cold saline infusion to increase malleability.[72–74] The effectiveness of clips is also limited by the size of the defect. Finally, clips may interfere with subsequent laparoscopic closure of defects.[75]

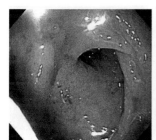 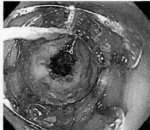 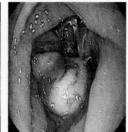

Fig. 4. Treatment of colocutaneous fistula in the sigmoid colon using an OTSC. Fistula in the sigmoid colon (*left*). Suction of fistula orifice into the OTSC cap (*middle*). Successful deployment of an OTSC and closure of fistula (*right*).

Table 2
Studies reporting efficacy of over-the-scope clips for fistulae and leak closure

Location	Study	Type of Clip	Number of Subjects	Short-Term Closure of Leak/Fistulae (%)
Upper GI tract	Kobara et al,[64] 2017	OTSC	44	82
	Law et al,[63] 2015	OTSC	34	85
	Mizrahi et al,[65] 2016	OTSC	30	66
	Mercky et al,[66] 2015	OTSC	19	89
	Niland & Brock,[67] 2017	OTSC	10	50
	Mennigen et al,[68] 2013	OTSC	9	89
Lower GI tract	Haito-Chavez et al,[69] 2014	OTSC	140	73 for leaks 43 for fistulas
	Mizrahi et al,[65] 2016	OTSC	21	33
	Arezzo et al,[70] 2012	OTSC	14	86
	Kobara et al,[64] 2017	OTSC	14	93
	Manta et al,[71] 2011	OTSC	11	92
	Law et al,[63] 2015	OTSC	11	91

SUTURES

The recent evolution of endoscopic suturing technology has allowed for full-thickness closure of GI luminal defects (**Fig. 5**). Closure of GI fistulae with sutures has been successfully demonstrated; however, it is technically more difficult than clip placement, requiring additional training and expertise.[76] However, endoscopic suturing provides the ability to close larger defects compared with clips. Similar to clips, suturing requires robust mucosa to hold the sutures when tissues are pulled in apposition.[6] Currently, endoscopic suturing is performed using the OverStitch device (Apollo Endosurgery, Austin, TX, USA), which is only compatible with a double channel therapeutic endoscope. A handle attaches to the hub of the endoscope and controls a metallic needle arm that attaches to the tip of the endoscope. These factors limit the utility of the device in areas such as the proximal colon or the small bowel.

In a retrospective series consisting of 71 subjects who underwent Roux-en-Y gastric bypass complicated by gastrogastric fistulae, 95% of the fistulae repaired with sutures had complete primary closure. However, recurrent fistula in the same location was found in 65% of these subjects after an average follow-up of 177 days. All of the fistulae that were greater than 20 mm before closure had reopened, whereas 32% of the fistulae that were less than 10 mm remained closed. Endoscopic closure of fistulae using sutures is technically feasible and safe; however, the

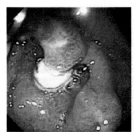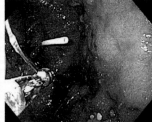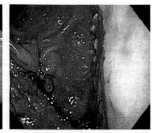

Fig. 5. Full-thickness endoscopic suturing of gastrocutaneous fistula after removal of a percutaneous endoscopic gastrostomy (PEG) tube. Fistula site (*left*). Suture being passed to the trocar using a biopsy forceps (*middle*). Complete closure of fistula with 2 interrupted sutures (*right*).

durability for larger fistulae may be limited based on these data. Endoscopic suturing is also useful for fixation of a covered SEMS (**Fig. 6**) and may significantly decrease the risk of migration.[40] Although endoscopic suturing is a technically feasible procedure, further study is needed to determine the long-term efficacy.

TISSUE ADHESIVE

One of the first successful closures of a fistula using fibrin glue was reported in 1990.[77] Fibrin glue and cyanoacrylate are tissue adhesives that can be used to seal GI defects. Cyanoacrylate has an advantage of stronger adhesion properties compared with fibrin glue. Cyanoacrylate's strong adhesion stems from its ability to polymerize after contact with anions, resulting in immediate polymerization on contact with GI tract tissue. Cyanoacrylates are not affected by gastric or pancreatic enzymes, making their use in the GI tract ideal.[78] In contrast, fibrin glue is most effective when applied to a dry area, making GI tract use more challenging.[79]

In a retrospective study of 52 subjects, only 55.7% of GI fistulae were successfully closed with application of fibrin glue. Of the fistulae that sustained complete closure, only 36.5% were treated with fibrin glue, whereas 23.1% required further surgical intervention.[80] In a smaller study of 15 subjects with GI fistula, complete closure of the fistula with fibrin glue was achieved in 86.6% of cases. Notably, 87.5% of the low-output fistulae achieved complete closure compared with 55% of the high-output fistulae.[81] Considering these findings, low-output fistulae may be more amenable to treatment with fibrin adhesive. However, data are limited and further study is required to corroborate this finding.

The efficacy of cyanoacrylate glue for closure of fistulae and leaks is well documented. A retrospective study by Kotzampassi and Eleftheriadis[78] evaluated 63 subjects with GI fistula treated with cyanoacrylate glue with a clinical success rate of 97%. A meta-analysis by Lopez and colleagues[82] reviewed 14 studies looking at the efficacy of cyanoacrylate in the closure of fistulae. The cumulative success rate in 203 subjects

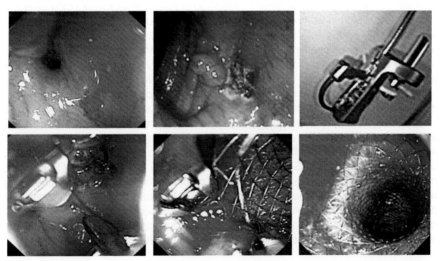

Fig. 6. Closure of ileal fistula. Ileal fistula (*upper left*). Argon plasma coagulation of fistula (*upper middle*). Tip of OverStitch device (*upper right*). Suturing closure of fistula (*lower left*). FCSEMS placement with suture fixation (*lower middle*). After closure with the FCSEMS (*lower right*).

was 81% with a 1% complication rate. The investigators agree that cyanoacrylate provided a feasible and safe intervention for fistulae and leaks. However, there is need for controlled prospective study to further validate these findings.

In addition to sealants, Vicryl (Ethicon Inc, Somerville [NJ]) mesh, and soft tissue grafts, such as Surgisis (Cook Surgical, Bloomington, IN, USA) made from the small intestinal submucosa of sheep, can be used to treat GI tract fistulae.[83] In a case series of 25 subjects with gastrocutaneous fistula, complete closure was achieved in 80%. Of the 20 cases that achieved complete closure, 1 application of Surgisis was needed in 30% of cases, 2 applications in 55%, and 3 applications in 15%.[84] For larger fistulae up to 30 mm in diameter, tissue adhesives can be applied in combination. Böhm and colleagues[85] reported promising results by combining the use of Vicryl mesh and fibrin glue. In this series, a Vicryl plug in combination with fibrin glue showed an 87% success rate in closure of fistulae.[85]

In addition to tissue adhesive combinations, there are multiple studies exploring the effectiveness of tissue adhesives combined with other endoscopic techniques for treatment of GI disruptions. One retrospective study looked at effectiveness of clips and glue versus surgical intervention. A total of 35 subjects with anastomotic leak underwent luminal repair with clips and fibrin glue or surgery. Technical success was achieved in 95% of the subjects undergoing endoscopic treatment, with clinical success in 100% of these cases. In the surgically treated group, 33% died due to sepsis, bleeding, or hospital-acquired pneumonia. Furthermore, endoscopic therapy resulted in a lower rate of leakage, 17.5%, compared with 58.3% with surgical treatment.[86] One small case series demonstrated successful closure of large diameter fistulae using fibrin glue and placement of a SEMS.[87]

Tissue adhesives play an important, yet evolving, role in treatment of GI tract fistulae. Currently, data are limited and further prospective studies will be key in determining the efficacy of these techniques and the potential advantages of combining adhesive therapy with other modalities.

COMPARISON OF DIFFERENT MODALITIES FOR FISTULA CLOSURE

One advantage of stents over other endoscopic interventions for fistula closure is the immediate protection of the defect, which allows for mucosal healing and early oral feeding.[47] However, stents possess their own set of limitations. For example, esophageal stents may be challenging to use for management of proximal esophageal lesions. In such situations clips may be used successfully.[88] **Table 3** summarizes the advantages and limitations of various endoscopic techniques for fistula closure.

There are a limited number of studies comparing efficacy of different endoscopic modalities for management of fistulae. One retrospective study compared the FCSEMS and the OTSC for repair of upper GI disruption. A total of 106 cases were reviewed with 69% treated with the FCSEMS and 31% treated with the OTSC. Clinical success after primary intervention was 40% for the FCSEMS and 70% for the OTSC with a P-value of 0.006. However, defects treated with an FCSEMS were larger than those treated with an OTSC (12.6. mm vs 7.1 mm). Furthermore, migration was a common complication for FCSEMS, with a rate up to 68%.[89] Given the retrospective nature of the study and disparity in size of lesions treated, it is not possible to determine superiority based on these data. With limited data comparing the efficacy of the different endoscopic techniques for fistula closure, the endoscopist must assess each individual case to choose the appropriate intervention.

RELATIONSHIP TO LUMEN APPOSING METAL STENTS

The LAMS was originally designed for drainage of pancreatic fluid collections. However, its use has been widely expanded to create iatrogenic fistula for therapeutic purposes.

Table 3
Comparison of different endoscopic modalities for gastrointestinal disruption repair

	Advantages	Disadvantages
Stents	Early oral intake Immediate protection Different compositions, delivery systems, covering for versatility	Migration Mandatory retrieval Difficult to use in lower GI defects
TTSC	Ease of use Rotatable Can be reopened	Require robust mucosa Reserved for smaller defects Limited grasping force Spontaneous dislodgement
OTSC	Higher grasping force than TTSC Larger clip size for larger defects Ease of use or setup	Require robust mucosa May limit subsequent laparoscopic closure of defect Difficult to remove
Sutures	Full-thickness plication Closure of larger defects	Requires robust mucosa Technically challenging and time consuming Difficult to use in proximal colon or small bowel
Tissue adhesive	May be used in combination with other modalities	Low success rate with high-output fistula

Aside from treatment of pancreatic collections, the LAMS has been used to perform choledochoduodenostomy for distal bile duct obstruction, gastrojejunostomy for gastroduodenal obstruction, cholecystoenterostomy for gallbladder drainage, drainage of pelvic or rectal fluid collections, and transgastric access in Roux-en-Y gastric bypass to allow for endoscopic retrograde cholangiopancreatography (ERCP).[90–94]

Removal of a LAMS after drainage of a pancreatic fluid collection is generally performed after 4 to 6 weeks. The removal interval of s LAMS after off-label use varies and data are limited. A primary concern after removal of a LAMS is a persistent fistula tract. The fistula tract will generally close spontaneously with resolution of the pancreatic collection. However, an application in which a persistent fistula tract is of concern is the creation of a transgastric fistula for performance of ERCP in Roux-en-Y gastric bypass because, theoretically, this causes weight gain. Creation of transgastric fistula with a LAMS has been reported in multiple studies. In these case series, the gastrogastric fistula was routinely closed using endoscopic suturing or an OTSC and weight gain was not reported. One case of persistent fistula was reported after closure with endoscopic suturing.[95] Further study is needed to determine the impact of persistent fistula after LAMS removal and whether closure of the fistula is necessary.

SUMMARY

GI fistulae and leaks are a significant cause of morbidity and mortality.[96,97] These defects may respond to initial conservative management, which entails nutritional support, treatment of infection, and reduction of fistula output. Many of these patients have undergone previous surgery and may have multiple comorbidities, making them poor candidates for surgical therapy. Endoscopic intervention offers a minimally invasive alternative modality. Endoscopic therapies currently available for treatment of fistulae and leaks include stenting, clipping, full-thickness suturing, and use of tissue adhesives. Although long-term clinically successful closure remains a challenge, techniques and technology continue to rapidly evolve. Further study is needed to establish the optimal techniques, including combination therapy for closure of GI fistula.

The advent of the LAMS has provided the endoscopist the ability to deliberately create a fistula to treat disease states. Currently, closure of defects after use of a LAMS is not considered routinely necessary. A LAMS should be left in place until a fistula tract has formed, to avoid perforation or leak. A residual fistula after removal of a LAMS may be undesirable in certain circumstances, such as transgastric ERCP in Roux-en-Y gastric bypass, because, theoretically, a persistent fistula may result in weight gain. Further study is essential to determine if residual fistula from a LAMS is a clinically significant issue and whether closure may be necessary in certain instances.

REFERENCES

1. Kumar N, Thompson CC. Endoscopic therapy for postoperative leaks and fistulae. Gastrointest Endosc Clin N Am 2013;23(1):123–36.
2. Falconi M, Pederzoli P. The relevance of gastrointestinal fistulae in clinical practice: a review. Gut 2001;49(Suppl 4):iv2–10.
3. Alexander ES, Weinberg S, Clark RA, et al. Fistulas and sinus tracts: radiographic evaluation, management, and outcome. Gastrointest Radiol 1982;7(2):135–40.
4. Kwon SH, Oh JH, Kim HJ, et al. Interventional management of gastrointestinal fistulas. Korean J Radiol 2008;9(6):541–9.
5. Gonzalez-Pinto I, Gonzalez EM. Optimising the treatment of upper gastrointestinal fistulae. Gut 2001;49(Suppl 4):iv22–31.
6. Willingham FF, Buscaglia JM. Endoscopic management of gastrointestinal leaks and fistulae. Clin Gastroenterol Hepatol 2015;13(10):1714–21.
7. Galie KL, Whitlow CB. Postoperative enterocutaneous fistula: when to reoperate and how to succeed. Clin Colon Rectal Surg 2006;19(4):237–46.
8. Reber HA, Roberts C, Way LW, et al. Management of external gastrointestinal fistulas. Ann Surg 1978;188(4):460–7.
9. Lynch AC, Delaney CP, Senagore AJ, et al. Clinical outcome and factors predictive of recurrence after enterocutaneous fistula surgery. Ann Surg 2004;240(5):825–31.
10. D'Harcour JB, Boverie JH, Dondelinger RF. Percutaneous management of enterocutaneous fistulas. AJR Am J Roentgenol 1996;167(1):33–8.
11. Kaur N, Minocha VR, Mundu M. Improving outcome in patients of high output small bowel fistula. Trop Gastroenterol 2004;25(2):92–5.
12. Makhdoom ZA, Komar MJ, Still CD. Nutrition and enterocutaneous fistulas. J Clin Gastroenterol 2000;31(3):195–204.
13. Fazio VW, Coutsoftides T, Steiger E. Factors influencing the outcome of treatment of small bowel cutaneous fistula. World J Surg 1983;7(4):481–8.
14. Berry SM, Fischer JE. Classification and pathophysiology of enterocutaneous fistulas. Surg Clin North Am 1996;76(5):1009–18.
15. di Costanzo J, Cano N, Martin J, et al. Treatment of external gastrointestinal fistulas by a combination of total parenteral nutrition and somatostatin. JPEN J Parenter Enteral Nutr 1987;11(5):465–70.
16. Yanar F, Yanar H. Nutritional support in patients with gastrointestinal fistula. Eur J Trauma Emerg Surg 2011;37(3):227.
17. Rombeau JL, Rolandelli RH. Enteral and parenteral nutrition in patients with enteric fistulas and short bowel syndrome. Surg Clin North Am 1987;67(3):551–71.

18. Coughlin S, Roth L, Lurati G, et al. Somatostatin analogues for the treatment of enterocutaneous fistulas: a systematic review and meta-analysis. World J Surg 2012;36(5):1016–29.

19. Martineau P, Shwed JA, Denis R. Is octreotide a new hope for enterocutaneous and external pancreatic fistulas closure? Am J Surg 1996;172(4):386–95.

20. Nubiola P, Badia JM, Martinez-Rodenas F, et al. Treatment of 27 postoperative enterocutaneous fistulas with the long half-life somatostatin analogue SMS 201-995. Ann Surg 1989;210(1):56–8.

21. Hernandez-Aranda JC, Gallo-Chico B, Flores-Ramírez LA, et al. Treatment of enterocutaneous fistula with or without octreotide and parenteral nutrition. Nutr Hosp 1996;11(4):226–9 [in Spanish].

22. Sancho JJ, di Costanzo J, Nubiola P, et al. Randomized double-blind placebo-controlled trial of early octreotide in patients with postoperative enterocutaneous fistula. Br J Surg 1995;82(5):638–41.

23. Scott NA, Finnegan S, Irving MH. Octreotide and postoperative enterocutaneous fistulae: a controlled prospective study. Acta Gastroenterol Belg 1993;56(3–4):266–70.

24. Torres AJ, Landa JI, Moreno-Azcoita M, et al. Somatostatin in the management of gastrointestinal fistulas. A multicenter trial. Arch Surg 1992;127(1):97–9 [discussion: 100].

25. Campos AC, Andrade DF, Campos GM, et al. A multivariate model to determine prognostic factors in gastrointestinal fistulas. J Am Coll Surg 1999;188(5):483–90.

26. Varadarajulu S, Banerjee S, Barth B, et al. Enteral stents. Gastrointest Endosc 2011;74(3):455–64.

27. Hunerbein M, Stroszczynski C, Moesta KT, et al. Treatment of thoracic anastomotic leaks after esophagectomy with self-expanding plastic stents. Ann Surg 2004;240(5):801–7.

28. Tokar JL, Banerjee S, Barth BA, et al. Drug-eluting/biodegradable stents. Gastrointest Endosc 2011;74(5):954–8.

29. Park JS, Jeong S, Lee DH. Recent advances in gastrointestinal stent development. Clin Endosc 2015;48(3):209–15.

30. Yim HB. Self-expanding metallic stents and self-expanding plastic stents in the palliation of malignant oesophageal dysphagia. Ann Palliat Med 2014;3(2):41–6.

31. Buscaglia JM, Ho S, Sethi A, et al. Fully covered self-expandable metal stents for benign esophageal disease: a multicenter retrospective case series of 31 patients. Gastrointest Endosc 2011;74(1):207–11.

32. Holm AN, de la Mora Levy JG, Gostout CJ, et al. Self-expanding plastic stents in treatment of benign esophageal conditions. Gastrointest Endosc 2008;67(1):20–5.

33. Langer FB, Wenzl E, Prager G, et al. Management of postoperative esophageal leaks with the Polyflex self-expanding covered plastic stent. Ann Thorac Surg 2005;79(2):398–403 [discussion: 404].

34. Dabizzi E, Arcidiacono PG. Update on enteral stents. Curr Treat Options Gastroenterol 2016;14(2):178–84.

35. Ishii K, Itoi T, Sofuni A, et al. Endoscopic removal and trimming of distal self-expandable metallic biliary stents. World J Gastroenterol 2011;17(21):2652–7.

36. Eubanks S, Edwards CA, Fearing NM, et al. Use of endoscopic stents to treat anastomotic complications after bariatric surgery. J Am Coll Surg 2008;206(5):935–8 [discussion: 938–9].

37. Bakken JC, Wong Kee Song LM, de Groen PC, et al. Use of a fully covered self-expandable metal stent for the treatment of benign esophageal diseases. Gastrointest Endosc 2010;72(4):712–20.

38. Eloubeidi MA, Talreja JP, Lopes TL, et al. Success and complications associated with placement of fully covered removable self-expandable metal stents for benign esophageal diseases (with videos). Gastrointest Endosc 2011;73(4):673–81.
39. Senousy BE, Gupte AR, Draganov PV, et al. Fully covered Alimaxx esophageal metal stents in the endoscopic treatment of benign esophageal diseases. Dig Dis Sci 2010;55(12):3399–403.
40. Law R, Prabhu A, Fujii-Lau L, et al. Stent migration following endoscopic suture fixation of esophageal self-expandable metal stents: a systematic review and meta-analysis. Surg Endosc 2017. [Epub ahead of print].
41. Mudumbi S, Velazquez-Aviña J, Neumann H, et al. Anchoring of self-expanding metal stents using the over-the-scope clip, and a technique for subsequent removal. Endoscopy 2014;46(12):1106–9.
42. van Halsema EE, van Hooft JE. Clinical outcomes of self-expandable stent placement for benign esophageal diseases: a pooled analysis of the literature. World J Gastrointest Endosc 2015;7(2):135–53.
43. Alazmi W, Al-Sabah S, Ali DA, et al. Treating sleeve gastrectomy leak with endoscopic stenting: the Kuwaiti experience and review of recent literature. Surg Endosc 2014;28(12):3425–8.
44. Swinnen J, Eisendrath P, Rigaux J, et al. Self-expandable metal stents for the treatment of benign upper GI leaks and perforations. Gastrointest Endosc 2011;73(5):890–9.
45. El Hajj II, Imperiale TF, Rex DK, et al. Treatment of esophageal leaks, fistulae, and perforations with temporary stents: evaluation of efficacy, adverse events, and factors associated with successful outcomes. Gastrointest Endosc 2014;79(4): 589–98.
46. Seven G, Irani S, Ross AS, et al. Partially versus fully covered self-expanding metal stents for benign and malignant esophageal conditions: a single center experience. Surg Endosc 2013;27(6):2185–92.
47. van Boeckel PG, Dua KS, Weusten BL, et al. Fully covered self-expandable metal stents (SEMS), partially covered SEMS and self-expandable plastic stents for the treatment of benign esophageal ruptures and anastomotic leaks. BMC Gastroenterol 2012;12:19.
48. Suzuki T, Siddiqui A, Taylor LJ, et al. Clinical outcomes, efficacy, and adverse events in patients undergoing esophageal stent placement for benign indications: a large multicenter study. J Clin Gastroenterol 2016;50(5):373–8.
49. Christophorou D, Valats JC, Funakoshi N, et al. Endoscopic treatment of fistula after sleeve gastrectomy: results of a multicenter retrospective study. Endoscopy 2015;47(11):988–96.
50. El Mourad H, Himpens J, Verhofstadt J. Stent treatment for fistula after obesity surgery: results in 47 consecutive patients. Surg Endosc 2013;27(3):808–16.
51. Eisendrath P, Cremer M, Himpens J, et al. Endotherapy including temporary stenting of fistulas of the upper gastrointestinal tract after laparoscopic bariatric surgery. Endoscopy 2007;39(7):625–30.
52. Salinas A, Baptista A, Santiago E, et al. Self-expandable metal stents to treat gastric leaks. Surg Obes Relat Dis 2006;2(5):570–2.
53. Garofalo F, Noreau-Nguyen M, Denis R, et al. Evolution of endoscopic treatment of sleeve gastrectomy leaks: from partially covered to long, fully covered stents. Surg Obes Relat Dis 2017;13(6):925–32.
54. Lamazza A, Sterpetti AV, De Cesare A, et al. Endoscopic placement of self-expanding stents in patients with symptomatic anastomotic leakage after colorectal resection for cancer: long-term results. Endoscopy 2015;47(3):270–2.

55. DiMaio CJ, Dorfman MP, Gardner GJ, et al. Covered esophageal self-expandable metal stents in the nonoperative management of postoperative colorectal anastomotic leaks. Gastrointest Endosc 2012;76(2):431–5.
56. Raju GS. Endoscopic clip closure of gastrointestinal perforations, fistulae, and leaks. Dig Endosc 2014;26(Suppl 1):95–104.
57. Rodella L, Laterza E, De Manzoni G, et al. Endoscopic clipping of anastomotic leakages in esophagogastric surgery. Endoscopy 1998;30(5):453–6.
58. Rustagi T, McCarty TR, Aslanian HR. Endoscopic treatment of gastrointestinal perforations, leaks, and fistulae. J Clin Gastroenterol 2015;49(10):804–9.
59. Kirschniak A, Kratt T, Stüker D, et al. A new endoscopic over-the-scope clip system for treatment of lesions and bleeding in the GI tract: first clinical experiences. Gastrointest Endosc 2007;66(1):162–7.
60. Matthes K, Jung Y, Kato M, et al. Efficacy of full-thickness GI perforation closure with a novel over-the-scope clip application device: an animal study. Gastrointest Endosc 2011;74(6):1369–75.
61. Monkemuller K, Peter S, Toshniwal J, et al. Multipurpose use of the 'bear claw' (over-the-scope-clip system) to treat endoluminal gastrointestinal disorders. Dig Endosc 2014;26(3):350–7.
62. Voermans RP, Le Moine O, von Renteln D, et al. Efficacy of endoscopic closure of acute perforations of the gastrointestinal tract. Clin Gastroenterol Hepatol 2012; 10(6):603–8.
63. Law R, Wong Kee Song LM, Irani S, et al. Immediate technical and delayed clinical outcome of fistula closure using an over-the-scope clip device. Surg Endosc 2015;29(7):1781–6.
64. Kobara H, Mori H, Fujihara S, et al. Outcomes of gastrointestinal defect closure with an over-the-scope clip system in a multicenter experience: an analysis of a successful suction method. World J Gastroenterol 2017;23(9):1645–56.
65. Mizrahi I, Eltawil R, Haim N, et al. The clinical utility of over-the-scope clip for the treatment of gastrointestinal defects. J Gastrointest Surg 2016;20(12):1942–9.
66. Mercky P, Gonzalez JM, Aimore Bonin E, et al. Usefulness of over-the-scope clipping system for closing digestive fistulas. Dig Endosc 2015;27(1):18–24.
67. Niland B, Brock A. Over-the-scope clip for endoscopic closure of gastrogastric fistulae. Surg Obes Relat Dis 2017;13(1):15–20.
68. Mennigen R, Colombo-Benkmann M, Senninger N, et al. Endoscopic closure of postoperative gastrointestinal leakages and fistulas with the over-the-scope clip (OTSC). J Gastrointest Surg 2013;17(6):1058–65.
69. Haito-Chavez Y, Law JK, Kratt T, et al. International multicenter experience with an over-the-scope clipping device for endoscopic management of GI defects (with video). Gastrointest Endosc 2014;80(4):610–22.
70. Arezzo A, Verra M, Reddavid R, et al. Efficacy of the over-the-scope clip (OTSC) for treatment of colorectal postsurgical leaks and fistulas. Surg Endosc 2012; 26(11):3330–3.
71. Manta R, Manno M, Bertani H, et al. Endoscopic treatment of gastrointestinal fistulas using an over-the-scope clip (OTSC) device: case series from a tertiary referral center. Endoscopy 2011;43(6):545–8.
72. Bauder M, Meier B, Caca K, et al. Endoscopic removal of over-the-scope clips: clinical experience with a bipolar cutting device. United European Gastroenterol J 2017;5(4):479–84.
73. Kapadia S, Nagula S, Kumta NA. Argon plasma coagulation for successful fragmentation and removal of an over-the-scope clip (OTSC). Dig Endosc 2017;29(7): 820–1.

74. Krishna SG, Shakhatreh M. Endoscopic removal of over-the-scope clip with cold saline solution technique. Gastrointest Endosc 2016;84(5):850–1.
75. Cho SB, Lee WS, Joo YE, et al. Therapeutic options for iatrogenic colon perforation: feasibility of endoscopic clip closure and predictors of the need for early surgery. Surg Endosc 2012;26(2):473–9.
76. Rajan E, Gostout CJ, Aimore Bonin E, et al. Endoscopic full-thickness biopsy of the gastric wall with defect closure by using an endoscopic suturing device: survival porcine study. Gastrointest Endosc 2012;76(5):1014–9.
77. Eleftheriadis E, Tzartinoglou E, Kotzampassi K, et al. Early endoscopic fibrin sealing of high-output postoperative enterocutaneous fistulas. Acta Chir Scand 1990; 156(9):625–8.
78. Kotzampassi K, Eleftheriadis E. Tissue sealants in endoscopic applications for anastomotic leakage during a 25-year period. Surgery 2015;157(1):79–86.
79. Rogalski P, Daniluk J, Baniukiewicz A, et al. Endoscopic management of gastrointestinal perforations, leaks and fistulas. World J Gastroenterol 2015;21(37): 10542–52.
80. Lippert E, Klebl FH, Schweller F, et al. Fibrin glue in the endoscopic treatment of fistulae and anastomotic leakages of the gastrointestinal tract. Int J Colorectal Dis 2011;26(3):303–11.
81. Rabago LR, Ventosa N, Castro JL, et al. Endoscopic treatment of postoperative fistulas resistant to conservative management using biological fibrin glue. Endoscopy 2002;34(8):632–8.
82. Lopez J, Rodriguez K, Targarona EM, et al. Systematic review of cyanoacrylate embolization for refractory gastrointestinal fistulae: a promising therapy. Surg Innov 2015;22(1):88–96.
83. Toussaint E, Eisendrath P, Kwan V, et al. Endoscopic treatment of postoperative enterocutaneous fistulas after bariatric surgery with the use of a fistula plug: report of five cases. Endoscopy 2009;41(6):560–3.
84. Maluf-Filho F, Hondo F, Halwan B, et al. Endoscopic treatment of Roux-en-Y gastric bypass-related gastrocutaneous fistulas using a novel biomaterial. Surg Endosc 2009;23(7):1541–5.
85. Böhm G, Mossdorf A, Klink C, et al. Treatment algorithm for postoperative upper gastrointestinal fistulas and leaks using combined vicryl plug and fibrin glue. Endoscopy 2010;42(7):599–602.
86. Lee S, Ahn JY, Jung HY, et al. Clinical outcomes of endoscopic and surgical management for postoperative upper gastrointestinal leakage. Surg Endosc 2013; 27(11):4232–40.
87. Victorzon M, Victorzon S, Peromaa-Haavisto P. Fibrin glue and stents in the treatment of gastrojejunal leaks after laparoscopic gastric bypass: a case series and review of the literature. Obes Surg 2013;23(10):1692–7.
88. Fischer A, Schrag HJ, Goos M, et al. Nonoperative treatment of four esophageal perforations with hemostatic clips. Dis Esophagus 2007;20(5):444–8.
89. Farnik H, Driller M, Kratt T, et al. Indication for 'Over the scope' (OTS)-clip vs. covered self-expanding metal stent (cSEMS) is unequal in upper gastrointestinal leakage: results from a retrospective head-to-head comparison. PLoS One 2015; 10(1):e0117483.
90. Irani S, Baron TH, Grimm IS, et al. EUS-guided gallbladder drainage with a lumen-apposing metal stent (with video). Gastrointest Endosc 2015;82(6):1110–5.
91. Ngamruengphong S, Nieto J, Kunda R, et al. Endoscopic ultrasound-guided creation of a transgastric fistula for the management of hepatobiliary disease in patients with Roux-en-Y gastric bypass. Endoscopy 2017;49(6):549–52.

92. Tsuchiya T, Bun Teoh AY, Itoi T, et al. Long-term outcomes of EUS-guided chole-dochoduodenostomy using a lumen-apposing metal stent for malignant distal biliary obstruction: a prospective multicenter study. Gastrointest Endosc 2017. [Epub ahead of print].

93. Tyberg A, Perez-Miranda M, Sanchez-Ocaña R, et al. Endoscopic ultrasound-guided gastrojejunostomy with a lumen-apposing metal stent: a multicenter, international experience. Endosc Int Open 2016;4(3):E276-81.

94. Manvar A, Karia K, Ho S. Endoscopic ultrasound-guided drainage of pelvic abscesses with lumen-apposing metal stents. Endosc Ultrasound 2017;6(4):217-8.

95. Kedia P, Tyberg A, Kumta NA, et al. EUS-directed transgastric ERCP for Roux-en-Y gastric bypass anatomy: a minimally invasive approach. Gastrointest Endosc 2015;82(3):560-5.

96. Ashkenazi I, Turégano-Fuentes F, Olsha O, et al. Treatment options in gastrointestinal cutaneous fistulas. Surg J (N Y) 2017;3(1):e25-31.

97. Takeshita N, Ho KY. Endoscopic closure for full-thickness gastrointestinal defects: available applications and emerging innovations. Clin Endosc 2016; 49(5):438-43.

How the Experts Do It: Step-by-Step Guide

Ji Young Bang, MD, MPH, Shyam Varadarajulu, MD*

KEYWORDS

- Lumen-apposing metal stent • Adverse events • Techniques • Challenges

KEY POINTS

- The development of lumen-apposing metal stents (LAMS) is a significant advancement in interventional EUS.
- The complexity of therapeutic EUS has been simplified as the LAMS enables better drainage via the wide lumen and facilitates access to adjacent structures to perform complex interventions.
- Further technical refinements are underway to expand the indications and further improve the safety profile of LAMS.
- In addition to evaluating clinical efficacy, well-designed randomized trials are required to study the cost-effectiveness of LAMS in patient management.

INTRODUCTION

It is postulated that lumen-apposing metal stents (LAMS) have 4 inherent advantages over traditional plastic stents. First, the large diameter (10–20 mm) facilitates better drainage of infective or necrotic contents. Second, the wider lumen can serve as a conduit to access structures adjacent to the gastrointestinal (GI) tract for performing interventions such as necrosectomy. Third, by the virtue of their ability to appose 2 adjacent structures, the LAMS likely minimize the risk of leakage. Fourth, LAMS are built on a single delivery platform that simplifies stent placement by reducing the number of procedural steps. Although there are 2 types of LAMS being used worldwide, their basic design and concept are quite similar (**Table 1**). Although the AXIOS stent is available in both a cautery- and noncautery-based delivery platform, the SPAXUS stent uses only a noncautery delivery system.

Center for Interventional Endoscopy, Florida Hospital, 601 East Rollins Street, Orlando, FL 32803, USA
* Corresponding author.
E-mail address: svaradarajulu@yahoo.com

Gastrointest Endoscopy Clin N Am 28 (2018) 251–260
https://doi.org/10.1016/j.giec.2017.11.011
1052-5157/18/© 2017 Elsevier Inc. All rights reserved.

Table 1
Currently available and widely used lumen-apposing metal stents

Company	Stent Name	Indication	Design Features
Boston Scientific	AXIOS	Endoscopic device to deliver a transenteric stent between the GI tract and a pseudocyst	• Proprietary one-step combined diathermic ring and cut-wire provides access into target tissue • MRI compatible, fully covered self-expanding metal stent is preloaded onto the delivery catheter • Perpendicular flanges secure tissue layers and help prevent migration • Large-diameter lumen (10–15 mm) apposition stent enables rapid, effective drainage, allowing passage of the endoscope through the stent for cystoscopy, irrigation, and debridement • Variable diameter (10, 15 mm) with 10 mm stent length
Taewoong Medical	SPAXUS	Drainage of pancreatic pseudocyst or gallbladder	• Lumen apposing design to prevent migration • Fully silicone-coated to prevent leakage and ingrowth • Flexible design accommodates apposition regardless of wall thickness • Variable diameter (8,10,16 mm) with 20 mm stent length • Wide and smooth flare edges to prevent migration and stent-related luminal damage

STENT PLACEMENT

Patient preparation prior to use of LAMS involves review of the patient's medical records, most recent imaging, and laboratory results in order to maximize technical and clinical success and minimize the risk of adverse events (**Box 1**).

Hot AXIOS

The Hot AXIOS stent and electrocautery-enhanced delivery system (Boston Scientific Corporation, Natick, Massachusetts) is a through-the-scope, fully covered self-expandable metal stent. After initial puncture using the electrocautery tip, the delivery catheter is advanced into the fluid collection or adjacent organ and the distal flange is deployed first under EUS guidance. The proximal flange is then released later under

> **Box 1**
> **Patient preparation prior to use of lumen-apposing metal stents**
>
> 1. Review the patient's medical records to confirm procedural indication.
> 2. Review cross-sectional imaging to ensure a safe window for drainage and exclude the presence of pseudoaneurysm in the vicinity of the WON.
> 3. Pertinent laboratory results such as INR and platelet count.
> 4. Intravenous prophylactic broad-spectrum antibiotics.

EUS guidance or endoscopic view (**Fig. 1**). Equipment preparation and a step-by-step guide to the deployment of the hot AXIOS stent are outlined in **Boxes 2** and **3** (see also **Fig. 2**).

The AXIOS stent is also available in a noncautery-based delivery system. After placing a 0.025/0.035-inch guidewire, the transmural tract is enlarged using cautery or a dilating balloon. This is followed by deployment of the AXIOS stent (over the guidewire) under EUS guidance.

SPAXUS

After puncturing the fluid collection or adjacent organ using a 19G needle, a 0.025/0.035-inch guidewire is advanced. The transmural tract is then dilated by application of cautery or using a balloon. The stent delivery catheter is then advanced over the guidewire, and the distal flange is first released, usually under fluoroscopic guidance. The delivery system is then gently pulled so that the distal flange is apposed to the wall of the GI tract. The proximal flange is then released within the GI lumen (**Fig. 3**).

TECHNICAL TIPS
Stent Deployment

Accessing a fluid collection using the electrocautery-enhanced tip can be technically challenging when the echoendoscope is acutely angulated. This is rarely encountered when attempting a puncture from the fundus/cardia of the stomach. Under such circumstances, the target is first accessed with a 19G needle, and a guidewire is coiled within it. The LAMS is then deployed over the guidewire as it provides safe anchorage.

Likewise, when a stent is placed at an anatomically difficult position, such as the gastric cardia or the second portion of the duodenum, deployment of the proximal

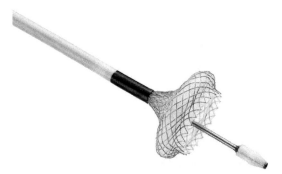

Fig. 1. The lumen-apposing Hot AXIOS stent (*Courtesy of* Boston Scientific, Marlborough, MA; with permission.)

Box 2
Equipment preparation

1. Remove the hot AXIOS stent with the electrocautery-enhanced delivery system from the package.
2. The delivery catheter is inserted into the working channel of the linear echoendoscope and then secured in place by tightening the luer lock.

---

flange under endoscopic view can be challenging, as visualization is suboptimal. Under such circumstances, the stent can be deployed within the working channel of the echoendoscope and then pushed out using the delivery catheter, simultaneously as the echoendoscope is being withdrawn.

Intraprocedural Stent Migration

Internal stent migration is encountered if the transmural tract is dilated excessively, when the proximal flange deployment is not adequately visualized, or when repeated entry is made via the lumen of stent, such as when performing endoscopic necrosectomy. Although most migrations can be managed by intubating the cavity/organ with the gastroscope and using rat-tooth forceps to retrieve the stent, in some instances the stent can migrate within a PFC that is not conducive for endoscopic intubation. In such instances, another LAMS can be deployed via the same tract. This facilitates ongoing drainage and minimizes the possibility of infection. The migrated stent can then be retrieved at later time by passing rat-tooth forceps via the lumen of the second stent and removing both stents at the same time. Another technique is to deploy a second LAMS within the lumen of the migrated stent. This may require guidewire

---

Box 3
Step-by-step guide to deployment of the hot AXIOS stent (see Fig. 2)

The delivery system of the hot AXIOS stent is numbered from 1 to 4 in order to guide the user during stent insertion and deployment. Numbers 1 and 3 apply to the catheter control portion of the delivery system (lower part of the handle) and numbers 2 and 4 apply to the stent deployment portion of the delivery system (upper part of the handle). The catheter control/stent deployment portion of the delivery system must be unlocked before and then locked after each step as applicable.

Step 1. Unlock the lower part of the delivery system. Push the lower part of the handle downwards while applying cautery in order to puncture the wall of the collection. Once the collection is punctured, lock the lower part of the delivery system.

Step 2. Remove the yellow safety clip from the gray-colored segment of the handle and unlock the stent deployment portion of delivery system. Pull the gray handle upwards halfway to release the distal flange of the LAMS. Deployment of the distal flange is performed under endosonographic view. When a click is felt, the deployment of distal flange is complete.

Step 3. Adjust the catheter control portion of the delivery system (lower part of the handle) so that under endoscopic view, the black mark is seen at the site where the catheter is entering the gastric/intestinal mucosa. Lock the catheter control portion of the delivery system.

Step 4. Pull the gray handle upwards to deploy the proximal flange of the LAMS under endoscopic view. Alternatively, the stent can be deployed within the working channel of the echoendoscope and then pushed out as the echoendoscope is being withdrawn.

Step 5. The delivery catheter is removed from the echoendoscope.

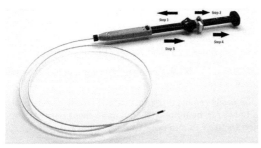

Fig. 2. Step-by-step guide to Hot AXIOS stent deployment. (*Courtesy of* Boston Scientific, Marlborough, MA; with permission.)

placement within the lumen of the index stent prior to deploying the second LAMS. The dumbbell flange of the second stent will lock the first LAMS, and when the second LAMS is pulled with biopsy forceps, both stents can be retrieved at the same time.

ADVERSE EVENTS
Immediate Bleeding

Bleeding can be encountered at the level of the mucosa or when intervening vasculature is traversed by the stent delivery system(**Box 4**). Mucosal bleeding can be stopped by local application of cautery in most patients. Intra-cystic/lesional hemorrhage can be visualized at sonography as hyperechoic spurting droplets (**Fig. 4**); when this is encountered, a guidewire can be advanced via the lumen of the stent delivery system, and the deployment hub is exchanged for a 19G FNA needle. The tip of the FNA needle is then positioned at the interface between cyst/organ and the GI tract wall layers, and epinephrine is gently injected until the bleeding stops. If bleeding persists and is significant, interventional radiology-guided coil placement may be required.

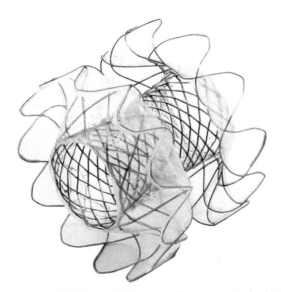

Fig. 3. The lumen-apposing SPAXUS stent (*Courtesy of* Taewoong Medical, Inc., Gyeonggi-do, South Korea; with permission.)

> **Box 4**
> **Postprocedure management**
>
> - CT or MRI scan is recommended in 3 weeks after drainage to assess treatment response.
> - If the collection has resolved, LAMS should be removed at 3 weeks after insertion to minimize stent-induced adverse events.
> - LAMS can usually be easily removed using standard biopsy or rat-tooth forceps. However, removal of buried LAMS can be more challenging; in these patients, the transmural tract may require dilation to 10 to 15 mm prior to stent removal.

Delayed Bleeding

Although late bleeding is mostly caused by underlying coagulopathy, LAMS-induced delayed bleeding has been recently reported.[1,2] Unlike plastic stents that gravitate toward the GI lumen as the PFC resolves, the LAMS remain in place with the resultant friction against regional vasculature surrounding the necrotic cavity precipitating bleeding (**Fig. 5**). Traditionally, a repeat CT or MRI is obtained at 6 to 8 weeks after intervention to assess treatment response, and the plastic stents are removed if the PFC has resolved. However, given the wider lumen of LAMS, PFCs tend to resolve faster. In a recent study,[1] delayed bleeding was observed after 3 weeks in several patients treated with LAMS, and in all cases, the PFCs had resolved completely. The authors therefore recommend obtaining a CT or MRI scan in 3 weeks to assess treatment response and to remove the stents if the PFC has resolved.

Buried Stents

In a recent case series of 2 patients who underwent LAMS placement for PFC and gallbladder drainage, buried stent syndrome was observed after 3 months.[3,4] Unlike the long, freely mobile plastic stents, LAMS are short and immobile. Therefore, following PFC resolution, the stent may become deeply embedded in the gastric wall layers with mucosal overgrowth. Removal of the buried stent can be technically challenging (**Fig. 6**). After widening the transmural tract up to 10 to 15 mm using a dilating balloon, the stent can be removed using wide-jaw biopsy forceps. However, this can be technically challenging and can result in bleeding. It is therefore important to remove the stents in a timely fashion once the fluid collection has resolved.

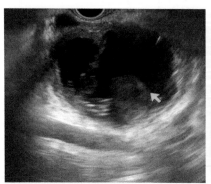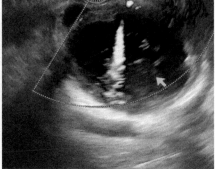

Fig. 4. Intra-cystic bleeding evidenced as hyperechoic spurt within the walled-off necrosis.

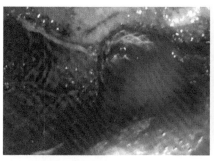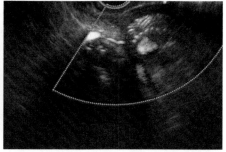

Fig. 5. Blood extruding via the LAMS and corresponding EUS image revealing vessels wrapping alongside the stent.

Biliary Obstruction

In patients undergoing transduodenal drainage of a PFC, once the fluid collection resolves, the distal flange of the LAMS can compress the distal common bile duct resulting in obstructive jaundice.[1] Removing the LAMS and placing a plastic stent in the bile duct will alleviate symptoms and result in stricture resolution (**Fig. 7**).

Delayed Stent Migration

LAMS can migrate within a cavity/organ or migrate externally into the gut lumen.[5] Internal migration may require intubation of the cavity using a diagnostic gastroscope for LAMS removal (using biopsy forceps). External migration of the LAMS can result in gastric outlet or intestinal obstruction (**Fig. 8**). Although most stents migrate spontaneously and can be managed by conservative measures, in persistently symptomatic patients with gastric outlet or intestinal obstruction, an upper or lower GI endoscopy may be required for stent retrieval.

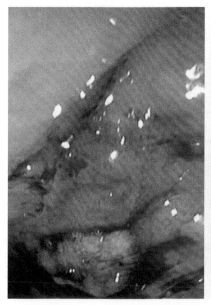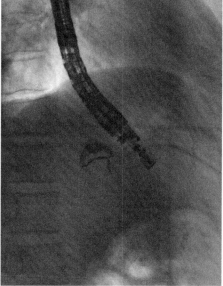

Fig. 6. LAMS buried underneath the gastric mucosa and visible only on fluoroscopy.

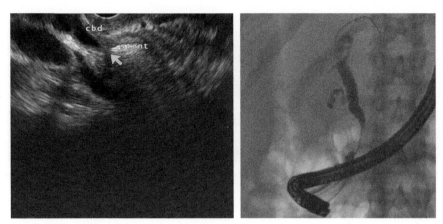

Fig. 7. LAMS compressing the distal bile duct and causing obstructive jaundice.

TREATMENT OUTCOMES
Pancreatic Fluid Collections

Most studies evaluating LAMS are retrospective, registry-based, case-control, or single-arm prospective series, and almost all studies appear to reach similar conclusions. One, the LAMS are technically easier to place than plastic stents with a shorter procedural duration.[6] Two, some studies have shown that the procedural duration for reinterventions (to perform necrosectomy/additional drainage) is also shorter in patients treated with LAMS as the necrotic cavity can be accessed without the need for additional dilation to perform necrosectomy.[7] Three, some studies observe that the rates of treatment success are higher and the number of reinterventions are fewer for patients treated with LAMS compared with plastic stents.[8] Four, although there

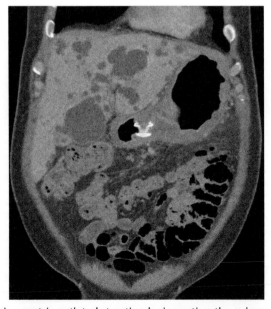

Fig. 8. LAMS causing gastric outlet obstruction by impacting the pylorus.

appears to be no difference in the rates of adverse events in patients treated with plastic versus LAMS, it is important to remove the LAMS in a timely manner to minimize stent-related adverse events. Lastly, LAMS are more expensive than plastic stents[6]; however, cost-effectiveness studies have not yet been conducted. Randomized trials comparing LAMS and plastic stents with outcomes focusing on reinterventions and costs are needed.

Other Interventions

Although outside the scope of this article, LAMS are now being used for other off-label indications such as gallbladder drainage, gastro-jejunal anastomosis, biliary ductal drainage, and for accessing the excluded stomach to perform ERCP in patients who have undergone gastric bypass surgery.

The technical and treatment success rates for gallbladder drainage exceed 90%, and the procedure is mostly performed in nonsurgical candidates.[9] Should cholecystectomy be undertaken at a later time, patients treated with LAMS may have to undergo an open surgery (not laparoscopy) given the creation of a large fistula in between the gallbladder and the stomach/duodenum. Gastro-jejunal anastomosis is being performed as an alternative technique to duodenal stent placement in patients with gastric outlet obstruction secondary to advanced malignancy.[10] Although experience is limited, a technical success rate of greater than 80% has been reported in expert hands. Small bowel peristalsis remains a challenge and appears to increase the risk of perforation and stent migration during deployment. Anchoring the small bowel using a balloon or T-tag facilitates the placement of LAMS via the stomach. Although EUS-guided biliary drainage is increasingly performed, the large-diameter LAMS (10–15 mm) are not suitable for placement in the common bile duct. Although small-diameter (6-8 mm) LAMS are being used in Europe for biliary ductal drainage, they are not available in the United States. Data on their clinical efficacy are not available at present. Finally, LAMS are being increasingly used for accessing the remnant stomach in patients with gastric bypass anatomy.[11] The LAMS are deployed via the gastric pouch, and the stents are left in situ for 2 to 3 weeks for the transmural tract to mature. A small-sized duodenoscope is then passed via the LAMS to access the major duodenal papilla. The LAMS is removed after treatment completion, and the fistulous tract closes spontaneously in more than 60% of patients. In patients with persistent fistula, the tract is closed using over-the-scope clips or by endoscopic suturing. Some experts recommend cauterizing the margins of the fistula with argon plasma coagulation to facilitate tissue growth and fistula closure.

SUMMARY

The development of LAMS is a significant advancement in interventional EUS. The complexity of therapeutic EUS has been simplified as the LAMS enables better drainage via the wide lumen and facilitates access to adjacent structures to perform complex interventions. Further technical refinements are underway to expand the indications and further improve the safety profile of LAMS. In addition to evaluating clinical efficacy, well-designed randomized trials are required to study the cost-effectiveness of LAMS in patient management.

REFERENCES

1. Bang JY, Hasan M, Navaneethan U, et al. Lumen-apposing metal stents (LAMS) for pancreatic fluid collection (PFC) drainage: may not be business as usual. Gut 2017;66(12):2054–6.

2. Lang GD, Fritz C, Bhat T, et al. EUS-guided drainage of peripancreatic fluid collections with lumen-apposing metal stents and plastic double-pigtail stents: comparison of efficacy and adverse event rates. Gastrointest Endosc 2018;87:150–7.
3. Fabbri C, Luigiano C, Marsico M, et al. A rare adverse event resulting from the use of a lumen-apposing metal stent for drainage of a pancreatic fluid collection: "the buried stent". Gastrointest Endosc 2015;82:585–7.
4. Rodrigues-Pinto E, Grimm IS, Baron TH. Removal of buried gastroduodenal stents after drainage of pancreatic fluid collections: silence of the LAMS (with video). Gastrointest Endosc 2016;83:853–4.
5. Dollhopf M, Larghi A, Will U, et al. EUS-guided gallbladder drainage in patients with acute cholecystitis and high surgical risk using an electrocautery-enhanced lumen-apposing metal stent device. Gastrointest Endosc 2017;86(4):636–43.
6. Bang JY, Hasan MK, Navaneethan U, et al. Lumen-apposing metal stents for drainage of pancreatic fluid collections: when and for whom? Dig Endosc 2017;29:83–90.
7. Mukai S, Itoi T, Baron TH, et al. Endoscopic ultrasound-guided placement of plastic vs. biflanged metal stents for therapy of walled-off necrosis: a retrospective single-center series. Endoscopy 2015;47:47–55.
8. Siddiqui AA, Kowalski TE, Loren DE, et al. Fully covered self-expanding metal stents versus lumen-apposing fully covered self-expanding metal stent versus plastic stents for endoscopic drainage of pancreatic walled-off necrosis: clinical outcomes and success. Gastrointest Endosc 2017;85:758–65.
9. Irani S, Ngamruengphong S, Teoh A, et al. Similar efficacies of endoscopic ultrasound gallbladder drainage with a lumen-apposing metal stent versus percutaneous transhepatic gallbladder drainage for acute cholecystitis. Clin Gastroenterol Hepatol 2017;15:738–45.
10. Itoi T, Ishii K, Ikeuchi N, et al. Prospective evaluation of endoscopic ultrasonography-guided double-balloon-occluded gastrojejunostomy bypass (EPASS) for malignant gastric outlet obstruction. Gut 2016;65:193–5.
11. Ngamruengphong S, Nieto J, Kunda R, et al. Endoscopic ultrasound-guided creation of a transgastric fistula for the management of hepatobiliary disease in patients with Roux-en-Y gastric bypass. Endoscopy 2017;49:549–52.

Printed and bound by CPI Group (UK) Ltd, Croydon, CR0 4YY

08/05/2025

01864711-0004